The Postnatal Depletion Cure

The Postnatal Depletion Cure

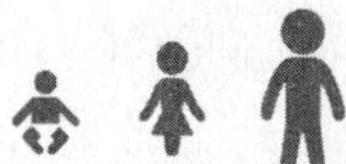

A COMPLETE GUIDE TO REBUILDING YOUR HEALTH AND RECLAIMING YOUR ENERGY FOR MOTHERS OF NEWBORNS, TODDLERS, AND YOUNG CHILDREN

Dr. Oscar Serrallach

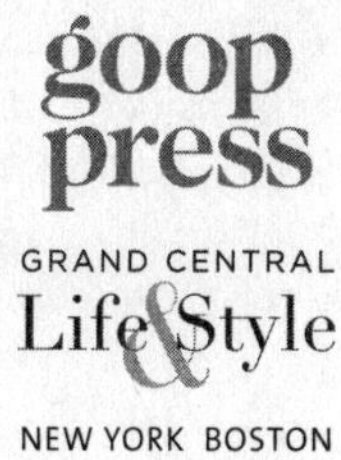

NEW YORK BOSTON

The advice herein is not intended to replace the services of trained health professionals or be a substitute for medical advice. You are advised to consult with your health-care professional with regard to matters relating to your health, and in particular regarding matters that may require diagnosis or medical attention.

Grand Central Life & Style
Hachette Book Group
1290 Avenue of the Americas, New York, NY 10104
www.GrandCentralLifeandStyle.com
www.goop.com

First Edition: June 2018

Grand Central Life & Style is an imprint of Grand Central Publishing. The Grand Central Life & Style name and logo are trademarks of Hachette Book Group, Inc.

The publisher is not responsible for websites (or their content) that are not owned by the publisher.

The Hachette Speakers Bureau provides a wide range of authors for speaking events. To find out more, go to www.hachettespeakersbureau.com or call (866) 376-6591.

Library of Congress Cataloging-in-Publication Data

Names: Serrallach, Oscar, author.
Title: The postnatal depletion cure: a complete guide to rebuilding your health and reclaiming your energy for mothers of newborns, toddlers, and young children / Dr. Oscar Serrallach.
Description: First edition. | New York: Grand Central Life & Style, 2018. | Includes bibliographical references.
Identifiers: LCCN 2017046606| ISBN 9781478970309 (hardcover edition) | ISBN 9781478970293 (ebook edition) | ISBN 9781478970590 (audio download)
Subjects: LCSH: Postnatal care—Popular works. | Postnatal care—Treatment—Popular works. | BISAC: HEALTH & FITNESS / Pregnancy & Childbirth. | FAMILY & RELATIONSHIPS / Parenting / Motherhood. | HEALTH & FITNESS / Women's Health. | HEALTH & FITNESS / Vitamins. | HEALTH & FITNESS / Healing.
Classification: LCC RG801 .S43 2018 | DDC 618.6—dc23
LC record available at https://lccn.loc.gov/2017046606

Printed in the United States of America

LSC-H

10 9 8 7 6 5 4 3 2 1

This book is dedicated to all mothers who have suffered and struggled in their selfless roles as caregivers, often without the unconditional support and wisdom from their culture, societies, and families that should have been their birthright. It is your strength that has inspired and guided me in writing this book.

The well-being of mothers is the fabric from which the cloth of the future of our society is made.

—Dr. Oscar Serrallach

Contents

PART III

THE SECOND AND THIRD TRIMESTERS: COMPLETING PHYSICAL RECOVERY

PART IV

RECOVERING YOUR LIFE

Introduction

I have written this book to answer a question many women ask: "How do I get my life and myself back after becoming a mother?" How do you find the strength to deal with your needs when our society tells us to focus entirely on the needs of the baby, causing you to disappear into the shadows of your predestined role? This infant-centered focus is something I witnessed in my practice as a doctor and as a father watching my extraordinary partner, Caroline, struggle after the birth of our children. It has been consistently mentioned by almost every mom I've spoken to, in contexts that vary from energy to illness to time management to self-confidence.

This is a *huge* hole in our thinking and treatment of new mothers. Worse, it's a hole that gets bigger and bigger because it's not discussed from a medical point of view. Postpartum depression, yes. Postnatal depletion? Say *what*? There's not even healthy dialogue around this concept, let alone healthy societal awareness and information.

What's just as, if not more, important to note is that postnatal depletion doesn't just affect new mothers—it affects *all* mothers. If a new mom isn't allowed to fully recover from the demanding requirements of pregnancy and birth, the aftereffects can last for *years*. I've treated women who were still depleted *ten years* after their babies were born. And if you then take into account the stress and sleeplessness associated with raising tweens and teenagers, coupled with the hormonal effects of perimenopause and menopause, it can become a pretty grim journey if mothers aren't truly supported and allowed to recover.

I know that this condition is real, and I know there is no need for you to suffer. There is almost a subconscious badge of honor associated with a mom's ability to juggle motherhood and child care with returning to work as soon as possible. Our Western culture has done mothers a great disservice by not honoring them on their road to recovery and giving them the time they need to adjust to the monumental changes in their lives. This needs to change! It is my hope that I can play a role in helping change the narrative of how we think about postpartum care, and it is urgent that we do. It was out of necessity that I went on a quest to help my darling partner, Caroline, back to health. But she helped me discover the reasons why mothers get so depleted, and what can be done to help them back to full functioning.

MY STORY

Nimbin is a small, quaint town about an hour's drive inland from Byron Bay, which is Australia's most eastern point in the state of New South Wales. I moved there in 2003, feeling unfulfilled as a doctor and needing a change to jolt me out of my career rut. I'd been a medical mercenary up until then, chasing jobs from city to city, working on everything from drug addiction to indigenous health to psychiatry to being part of the Emergency Department team in the coastal town of Ballina.

Unlike most other areas of medicine, emergency medicine is uncompromisingly simple: patients have specific needs that we can treat on the spot. I really enjoyed the camaraderie, and my schedule left me time to learn how to surf, practice my guitar, and be a player-coach for my local soccer club. But a deep restlessness and frustration led me to Nimbin, a town renowned for being a center of counterculture in my country; even though I didn't buy into the town's somewhat notorious hippie ethos of "free love and drugs," I dove into the deep ecological consciousness that was also an integral part of living in this area. I met many inspiring people with thought-provoking ideas. This is where my evolution as a doctor began.

At a music festival in 2003, I met Caroline Cowley, who soon became my life partner. Although she was a high-flying professional, born and bred in the metropolitan city of Melbourne, I was able to convince her to come live in the sleepy countryside surrounding Nimbin. We fell deeply in love and got very caught up in the romantic idealism of self-sufficiency. We created a thriving garden and spent many hours working on the land. It became quickly apparent to us that in this idyllic scenario we wanted to start a family, which led us to become involved in the thriving local home-birth community.

Having been trained in orthodox medicine, it was not an easy thing for me to embrace the idea of our first child being born outside a hospital setting. It took many meetings with home-birthing moms, experienced midwives, and doctors who'd had home births with their own children to finally warm me up to the idea. I tapped into an incredible amount of support and information about prenatal and postpartum care, from books, workshops, and mothers we met. One of the most wonderful experiences was when Caroline had a "blessingway ceremony"—a tradition in the Native American culture in which the mothers sit in a circle and share stories in support of the mother-to-be. As the father-to-be, I was taken on a ceremonial walk by an aboriginal friend of mine to a sacred area to celebrate my up-and-coming role. It was a beautiful experience and made me feel part of the long, ancient history of generations birthing generations. Still, I couldn't help myself: I wrote a very detailed birth plan in case we did need to make the transfer to hospital!

Caroline and I were very fortunate to have a beautiful and totally routine home birth with our first child, Felix, surrounded by family and loved ones. Our local community even organized a meal-delivery roster for a full two weeks, so we didn't have to think about what to cook when we were sleep deprived and adjusting to our amazing little baby. The instant quagmire of parenting left us overwhelmed with decisions. Do we use cloth diapers or disposables? Should we use a pacifier? How long should Caroline breastfeed? Why was the baby crying? As any parent will tell you, as soon as you answer one question, a new one arises—as do the judgments and criticisms (however well intended) of friends, loved ones, and, of course, all those "well-meaning" strangers.

A similar pattern occurred with our next two children, Maximo and Olivia. Caroline became more and more exhausted with each new baby, and we reached a crisis point soon after the birth of our third child, Olivia. Caroline's memory and concentration were shot. She felt as if she were drowning in her own sense of overwhelm, she had constant brain fog (commonly called baby brain), she suffered from a loss of confidence and a feeling of isolation, and she was not able to take care of herself fully. She was extremely fatigued, suffered anxiety, felt her sleep was superficial at best, and had a deep fear that she was never going to recover.

As my worries about my wife deepened with each passing day, I remembered a patient I'd had when I first started working at the Nimbin Medical Centre—a gaunt mother named Susan. In her midtwenties, she already had five young children, and not surprisingly she was exhausted and finding it difficult to cope. She was extremely anxious during our appointment, and it was hard for her to describe exactly what was bothering her and how she was feeling, aside from general stress and utter fatigue. I was concerned and wanted to do everything that I could to help her. I ordered blood tests to make sure she wasn't anemic and did a postpartum-depression screening test. I helped her arrange a social-worker appointment and a community-nurse home visit. When the blood work came back showing that she had low levels of iron, we discussed how this would have been contributing to her fatigue. We looked at ways of increasing iron in her diet while starting a simple iron supplement. Susan came in for her next appointment and I gently suggested that a referral to a counselor or psychologist might help her feel a lot better. I was just starting to pat myself on the back for a job well done and for going the extra mile for someone obviously in need—especially as my appointments with Susan always took closer to forty-five minutes than the usual twenty I was allotted—when she suddenly stood up and said, "God, I have to go." She grabbed her handbag and ran out the door before I could say a word.

The next week I followed up with the community nurse who had visited Susan at home. The nurse told me that Susan was feeling a little bit better and did not require our services. I was very surprised. I couldn't shake thinking about how Susan had seemed so distraught, running on empty, when I'd seen her.

Nearly eighteen months went by before I saw Susan again—this time in the ER of our local hospital with a bad case of pneumonia. She'd had another child by then and looked as exhausted and stressed-out as the first time I'd seen her. I admitted her to the hospital early in the morning to administer intravenous antibiotics, yet by late afternoon she stated that she was feeling better and was adamant that she had to go home. The meds had barely started to work, and she was discharged against medical advice. I haven't been able to find out what happened to her and her family, and I still wonder about her and worry how she's doing.

Desperate by this point to help Caroline on her road to recovery, I'd been keeping copious notes about my patients. I thought of other mothers I had seen—not all of them with symptoms as extreme as Susan's, but with similar issues. They were mothers like my own partner, who was, I realized, far from unique in her suffering. These moms loved their children. But they were also miserable and completely drained. They were not themselves and seemed to have given up hope that they might ever recover their vitality. What if all my patients with similar, recurring symptoms had the same condition? What if the physical depletion caused by the demands of their pregnancies started a cascade effect of all these other things that left them exhausted, anxious, and miserable?

With the notion of postnatal depletion fueling me, I realized there was a pattern—something I could investigate. I started to trawl through the medical literature and textbooks, and I was speechless to find that almost nothing had been written about what seemed to be such an incredibly important topic. All I could uncover was information on postnatal depression and some small-scale studies looking at postnatal fatigue. Caring for the baby was the dominant topic. Completely overlooked were the moms needing care for themselves so that they could best care for their babies, and there was in fact nothing at all about postnatal depletion.

It was a lightbulb moment. I began to look outside of Western medicine for ideas on how to better support a mother's needs after she gives birth. I read about the ancient wisdom of many indigenous cultures in which the time for mothers to fully recuperate was deeply respected and etched into the very social fabric of these cultures. These new mothers were supported by others in their community during this time of recovery: they were allowed to regain their strength, rest, and recuperate while bonding with their newborns. In our society, however, the typical dialogue tends to revolve around when the mother is going back to work and not much else.

I have no doubt that nearly all moms—no matter when they gave birth—can fully recover from postnatal depletion, regaining health and wellness far beyond what they have experienced in the past. I have seen the recovery process firsthand. With this book, I hope to give you the tools you need to restore your energy and sense of well-being.

HOW TO USE THIS BOOK

The book is divided into four easy-to-use parts:

- In part 1, "Defining Postnatal Depletion," I explain the causes of postnatal depletion and provide details about the physical, mental, and emotional conditions it creates, as well as why these conditions occur and can worsen during pregnancy and following birth. I also identify specific symptoms associated with postnatal depletion, giving you an understanding from a medical point of view about why you're feeling so lethargic and unlike yourself, and I describe how non-Western cultures treat the postnatal period. There's an awful lot of wonderful wisdom in how these societies regard and support new moms.
- In part 2, "One Hundred Days of Repletion: Rebuilding Physical Wellness," I describe how to replace vital micronutrients and macronutrients that will help your body recuperate. I also discuss how to rebuild your hormones and your energy and how to get the deep, sound sleep you really, really need!

- In part 3, "The Second and Third Trimesters: Completing Physical Recovery," I also tell you exactly what to eat and when for optimal nourishment. This will not only diminish your depletion, but, if you're breastfeeding, give your baby the ample rewards of your nutritious and delicious eating. In addition to this food plan, I also offer you a structured exercise/movement plan that is gentle and simple and costs you nothing. Without your even realizing it, these plans will help you lose the baby weight in the healthiest way possible.
- In part 4, "Recovering Your Life," I show you how to focus on your emotional well-being, get your libido back, and improve all your important relationships. I also give you the information you need to set up your home and environment in a way that better supports your health in the long term.
- The appendixes give you an accelerated recovery plan should you need to return to work, along with recipes, meal plans, and resources.

Through my own experiences as a father and husband, and in my professional work in integrative care, I have devoted my career to the treatment of postnatal depletion. Now, nearly a decade after I first started researching this phenomenon in earnest, I've written this book to give all moms (and their loved ones) the vital information they need to understand what will happen to their bodies, minds, and souls before, during, and after pregnancy. My goal is to give you the hope and support you deserve and to ease your worries—especially if you are feeling hopeless, as my partner once did. I'm going to give you all the tools you need to speed up your recovery and leave you feeling stronger, happier, and fully engaged with your baby and everyone else in your life. Your body has created a miracle, so let me show you how to find your way back to a full recovery.

PART I

Defining Postnatal Depletion

CHAPTER 1

What Is Postnatal Depletion?

Having a baby is one of the greatest joys a woman can experience. Making a new life is miraculous, life changing, and monumental. Seeing your baby's face for the first time is a wonderfully loving moment like no other.

Yet this magical life change can also create a perfect storm to destabilize a woman's psyche. I've seen so many women go from highly functioning, world-traveling, happily ambitious, contented, emotionally centered, and utterly competent and organized professionals to zombie-like diaper-changing milking machines practically overnight. As you know, the physical act of nurturing a baby inside your body requires a huge amount of resources. Your body is designed to give that baby everything he or she needs to make it to term—often at your expense. This is due to the incredible ability of the placenta, through intriguingly complex mechanisms, to coerce and then extract what it needs from the mother.

And then, when it's time for the baby to be born, the physical act of delivery also takes its toll—that's why it's called *labor*! You might not know that it's very common to lose blood during an uncomplicated vaginal delivery; the average amount is about 17 ounces—more than 2 cups!—which is about what you would be allowed to donate at a blood bank. The average amount of blood loss for an uncomplicated cesarean birth is approximately twice that, at 34 ounces.

If you're breastfeeding, the process might be satisfying, especially as you know your baby is getting proper nourishment, but it is also taxing due to the caloric and specific nutrient demands put on your body that making breast milk entails. Add into the mix ongoing sleep deprivation, the preset expectation of self-sufficiency that society has conditioned you to believe (think "I can do it all" and "My baby will never cry"), unending and repetitive chores, a body that feels forever changed, an often-hurried diet, and a total change of life direction.

Enter the well-meaning yet unhelpful comments, critiques, and endless comparisons to your friends' and family members' perfect little sleepers, who latched on to the breast without a peep (while your nipples are so sore you think they're about to explode), and early motherhood can begin to feel much more like a gauntlet to survive than a rewarding experience to enjoy.

WHAT EXACTLY IS POSTNATAL DEPLETION?

Postnatal depletion is a constellation of symptoms affecting all spheres of a mother's life after she gives birth. These symptoms arise from physiological issues, hormonal changes, and interruption of the circadian day/night rhythm of her sleep cycle, layered with psychological, mental, and emotional components.

Think of your body as a plastic bag full of water. The more water in the bag, the better you feel and the better you are able to cope. Each day of pregnancy, the birth, each sleepless night, each long day of breastfeeding, is like putting tiny pinpricks in the plastic bag. You can repair these holes, but it takes a little time. When there are only a few sticks of the pin, only a very small amount of water escapes the bag. The trouble, though, is when the holes start to come more quickly than you can repair them. Such is the body after childbirth; when there are too many stressors and not enough time to recover, your levels become depleted. Depending on the severity of depletion, the postnatal period can last for *years* after the baby is born—you can be left with a bag so filled with holes that it takes a long time to repair and refill. In the worst-case scenarios, I've even seen the depletion pattern occurring *decades* later. None of this suffering should continue for so long!

At its core, postnatal depletion is the understandable outcome of a series of less-than-ideal events leading to depletion of a woman's well-being at multiple levels. There are three primary factors at play here:

1. The nutrients given over to making, incubating, and birthing the baby are enormous, and this depletion continues after the birth for women who are breastfeeding.
2. Bone-gnawing exhaustion can occur from sleep deprivation—the result of never having a good, refreshing night's sleep.
3. The drastic change of a new mother's role is often accompanied by social isolation, which can have a deleterious effect on a woman's psychological well-being.

Postnatal Depletion Is a Syndrome

In my many years of studying postnatal depletion, I've found incredibly few texts written about it. It's important to understand why, because in order to get the best treatment, you're going to have to think outside the box, as I have learned to do.

I view postnatal depletion as a spectrum on a scale from mild and moderate to severe. I view postpartum depression as a separate condition, but with a strong overlap of symptoms and issues with postnatal depletion. There are two important points that differentiate them. Postpartum depression is marked by true clinical depression that is pervasive, and it is also marked by "anhedonia," which is a state in which a person takes no pleasure or joy from a situation or experience that in the past would have given them pleasure or joy. (Having a much-wanted baby is obviously that kind of situation.) Postpartum depression can be dangerous and must be treated by trained and competent mental-health professionals.

With postnatal depletion, I realized I needed to push past my medical school training and find a better system than the linear-thinking model, because my patients were suffering and my conventional treatments weren't working. The linear-thinking model, on which conventional modern medicine is based, posits that cause A leads to effect B. In this model, effect B can be caused only by cause A. There is no other explanation. I'm sure you've dealt with this situation if you've ever gone to a doctor with certain symptoms, only to have them dismissed because they weren't "typical."

Try thinking of a room as a set of symptoms and signs that someone may typically experience with a disorder or a condition. When there is only one door into that room (such as cause A leading to effect B; for example, you have hypertension or high blood pressure, leading to damage in your arteries related to plaque buildup and a subsequent higher risk of strokes and heart attacks), that room is called a *disease.* Modern medicine does an excellent job of dealing with diseases. A *syndrome*, however, is a set of commonly experienced symptoms usually caused by many different factors—this would be as if the room had many doors into it, and it was not immediately clear which door led you into the room or set of symptoms.

Western medical doctors tend not to like syndromes because the linear-thinking model is too simplistic for effective treatment. But that's what postnatal depletion is.

Postnatal depletion also involves many mineral, vitamin, and nutrient *insufficiencies*; a disease process typically deals with a *deficiency.* It's important to understand the difference between these two words. Insufficiency is where the level of a mineral, vitamin, or nutrient is not in the disease-producing range, but in the suboptimal range. In other words, an insufficiency won't give you a disease, but it means that your cells and organs are not able to run properly. This, in turn, can make you feel terrible.

POSTNATAL DEPLETION FACTORS

Before motherhood, the typical modern woman with her busy, high-paced life is usually already close to the maximum capacity of what she and her body can handle. Conception and pregnancy require huge amounts of physical resources, and then the baby's delivery (whether by cesarean or vaginal delivery) places further strain on these physical resources—and this is just day one of being a mother! Breastfeeding or bottle-feeding a baby requires more precious resources; the average child needs 1 million calories of food before he or she is independent. Throw sleep deprivation into the mix, and it's no surprise that moms can feel overwhelmed, overworked, overstimulated, and overneeded.

In our society, the time and resource demands of motherhood are higher than ever. And unfortunately, it's becoming increasingly difficult for parents to easily access the nonhired help of family and community to assist in looking after children. This mismatch between expectation and support, stacked on top of nutrient depletion, leads directly to mothers feeling overwhelmed A new mother's biology is not designed and shouldn't be expected to have to deal with this level of ongoing and constant demands.

In my clinic, I do not see mothers who have failed or who are not trying hard enough. What I do see every day are mothers who are physically and emotionally depleted, exhausted, and stressed. They are at the end of their tether with no relief in sight.

Let's take a deeper look at the four main factors causing postnatal depletion.

Stress Factors

As a modern mom, whether a wife, partner, or single, you know all about stress. You've likely spent years building a satisfying career, but even with help from your partner, you still need to shop and cook and clean and budget and get a new muffler for the car. You want to make time for your friends and loved ones, and you long to find a few minutes for yourself every day. You might have delayed motherhood due to the need to work or other financial considerations. This is a fairly recent trend; the average age in Australia of a mother having her first baby is 30.9 years. In the United States, according to the Centers for Disease Control and Prevention (CDC), the average age is 26.3. How can you *not* feel vulnerable? Maybe you don't have a very family-friendly job and are allowed no more than a few weeks of parental leave, so you're already worried about how to pay for child care. Yep, you're stressed... and then along comes baby!

Motherhood is messy business; changing endless dirty diapers and washing baby puke out of your favorite shirt is humbling. How can you not be stressed when the baby is feeding what seems like 24/7 and you haven't slept properly in a month? This is compounded by physical stressors: your body has been taxed by pregnancy and childbirth, by the demands of breastfeeding, by sleep deprivation, and by all the other demands associated with caring for another human being. Also, if you've had your baby later in life, the stress can be even more difficult to manage because you've had more time to establish your own routines, which are now being radically overhauled by your little one.

Social Factors

From a medical point of view, the focus on postpartum care is almost always on the needs of the baby, not the mother—unless the mother is showing signs of serious postpartum depression.

I see this happen all the time at the medical centers where I work, at parents' groups, at child-care centers, with friends and families of friends, and in our general community. One of the strangest things that struck me was an unspoken *competitiveness*, which stemmed not so much from new parents but from society in general.

Take the birth itself. After the ordeal of childbirth, a message is sent out to the world stating the arrival of the baby and broadcasting the length of labor, the drugs used (or not), and the baby's weight and gender. (If you're really lucky, you'll be told what the Apgar score is, too!) "Mother and baby are doing well" is the typical message. But that is the last time *mother* shows up in the same sentence as *baby*. This begins what is potentially an unhealthy dialogue in which intense focus on the baby is accompanied by a decided lack of pragmatic and emotional support for the baby's mother.

The reality of modern parents is that the first time they are deeply involved in looking after a child is usually with their own baby. This is so common that we don't even think about it, but that's really a crazy fact! It's like driving a car for the first time in rush-hour traffic without ever having taken lessons or receiving a license—and with no road map provided. For many people, parenting is an abstract concept—until it's 3:00 a.m. and they're holding an actual screaming baby who won't settle down no matter what, leaving them delirious with exhaustion. From a social perspective, the only feedback that a new mother is likely to get is in the form of cultural values, competitiveness, and conflicting advice from other "parental drivers." This is a guaranteed recipe for self-doubt and parental anxiety.

This self-doubt can often manifest in what I call the phenomenon of choice overload. Most parents want the best for their children, making them an advertiser's or a marketer's dream. Which stroller is the best? Is it okay to buy something more affordable than the top-rated car seat? Is baby's bottom going to chafe without those brand-name wipes and a wipes warmer? What about the crib? Welcome to our brave new world of mommy-and-daddy consumerism, where the pressure to find the "best" products and the "right" routine can be crippling.

Pregnancy is an exciting but stressful time for so many women, particularly for those who struggled to get pregnant in the first place. That struggle makes it all the more painful when motherhood is taxing. Many women worry that if it's not all joy, if they don't have an instant instinct for tending to their child's every need, then they are failing somehow. Factor in the fears that they're also letting down the woman they used to be and that they're feeling unprepared for the tasks at hand, and their sense of inadequacy becomes palpable. Vulnerable new moms may also be subjected to judgment from their inner circle, a group that may consist of well-intentioned other mothers, mothers-in-law, sisters, aunts, other family members, neighbors, friends, and colleagues. The baby isn't gaining weight or is having trouble eating? It's probably because Mom's doing something wrong. Who's responsible if the baby isn't sleeping well or has colic? Mommy, of course. These judgments aren't always said aloud, but they're implied by silence, subtle eye rolls, or offers of myriad suggestions that worked for someone else.

If this kind of undermining comes from your beloved partner, it can be even more devastating. A shell-shocked and exhausted partner can inadvertently make things much worse. A change in a once-happy established dynamic can send even the best and sturdiest relationships into a downward spiral. (For much more on this topic, see chapter 13.)

Shaming, whether subtle or overt, can have devastating consequences. This is even more reason why expectant and new parents need so much support and why we need to open up a healthy dialogue about realistic expectations and care.

Predisposing Physical Factors, Primarily Inflammation

Predisposing factors that impact your physical and mental health also make you more vulnerable to experiencing postnatal depletion. Being an older mother, for example, is a predisposing factor due solely to physiology, as older women take longer to recover from major events such as childbirth, are more sensitive to the negative effects of sleep deprivation, and have hormones that are harder to regulate.

Physiologically, inflammation is the key hallmark and consequence of postnatal depletion. It also exacerbates and sometimes causes depletion's typical symptoms, as well as perpetuates the problem. In other words, inflammation begets inflammation.

There are many different types of inflammation, but at its core, inflammation occurs when there is either repairing or rebuilding going on in your body, or too many pro-oxidants being produced. Pro-oxidants are the harmful by-product of metabolic processes like oxygen consumption, and the clearing of toxic substances such as pesticides or cosmetics from the body. Pro-oxidants do have a role where they help stimulate the immune system and the detoxification systems of the body—it is all about balance. I picture a pro-oxidant like a bill or debt, and antioxidants are like the cash or check that will help clear that bill. In the world of finance, economists know that for a healthy economy you need a good balance of buying and selling, and if this is out of balance it contributes to inflation. In the body this inflation contributes to inflammation.

Inflammation in and of itself is not bad, but too much certainly is; just as a society with too high a rate of inflation suffers, a body with too much inflammation also suffers.

A major cause of inflammation is found in your gut. Not for nothing is your gut called the second brain. It is one of the most important regulators of inflammation in your body, if not *the* most important one. Your microbiome—the healthy and unhealthy bacteria that process your food—can make you (and keep you healthy), but it can break you (make you sick), too.

Environmental Factors

One of the biggest predisposing factors for postnatal depletion is environmental toxins. *Toxin* is one of those buzzwords that is casually thrown around by people even though they might not know what it actually means. A toxin is essentially a substance that causes some part of the body to react in a negative way. Technically, toxins are produced only by living things, but the term is loosely used here to include other substances, such as heavy metals, air pollution from traffic, and some personal-care products. You may be surprised to know that *we* produce most toxins, within our bodies; these are called *endogenous* toxins. These toxins are created during digestion and when your body burns oxygen to provide energy. The by-products of the oxygen burn are unstable molecules called free radicals. Your homemade toxins are totally normal, and your body is programmed to handle them so that they don't have a toxic effect. In fact, these endogenous toxins are absolutely necessary for waking up and stimulating our antioxidant systems and the cleansing pathways within the body.

The issue lies with your personal load of *exogenous* toxins, those produced outside the body, and whether they are having a toxic effect on your body. Exogenous toxins enter your system when you eat or drink them (e.g., foods containing pesticide or herbicide residue), breathe them (e.g., exhaust fumes or other pollution), or absorb them (e.g., cosmic radiation and ultraviolet rays from the sun and cleansing or personal-care products with harsh chemicals).

Your body is good at processing and eliminating endogenous toxins, but it is not efficient at clearing exogenous toxins, which usually require a lot of energy and resources to get out of your system.

If we overload that system, the toxic load can take hours to clear, which is why you might feel okay after a small amount of alcohol but experience the dreaded hangover after consuming more alcohol than your body can process. Your body is constantly processing toxins and may be having small hangover-like events all through the day or night... leading to brain fog, lethargy, muscle soreness, sugar cravings, and sleep problems.

The more toxins you are exposed to, the more inflammation they will create, which means the longer your recovery time will be because you'll be far less resilient to stress. If you used to recover relatively quickly from a bad night's sleep, you'll find it much more difficult to do so if suffering from inflammation triggered by postnatal depletion.

A developing fetus tends to be very sensitive to toxins. This is why your obstetrician likely offered restrictions on what you should do or eat while pregnant. On the toxin list will be cigarettes, alcohol, raw cheeses, fish high in mercury (like sushi tuna or swordfish), and extreme heat (such as a sauna or hot tub). It's often with much alarm and horror that pregnant moms learn just how these toxins may be affecting their baby. So many moms have told me about their deep guilt, shame, and worries that they may have unwittingly exposed their precious fetuses—as well as their own bodies—to the potentially damaging effects of pollutants and toxins. The problem is that these restrictions aren't based on rigorous science but merely on common sense. We simply do not know the facts for certain, mainly because it is ethically impossible to do any testing on pregnant women; you can't do a study in which some pregnant women are asked to eat a lot of tuna, for example, as it may cause harm.

In my practice, I often see women who start questioning their bodies, their own intuition, their food choices, their habits (good and bad), and even the quality of information that they get from all different sources—some excellent, some bogus and harmful. This, combined with the severe fatigue and baby brain that often accompany postnatal depletion, is a recipe for a downward spiral.

This downward spiral leads to the feelings of ongoing overwhelm and has undesirable effects on all aspects of a mother's functioning and well-being.

WHY POSTNATAL DEPLETION IS SO COMMON IN WESTERN SOCIETIES

When I started researching postnatal depletion patterns, trying to understand how and why it was happening to so many of my patients, I knew I had to push past just reading medical textbooks. Postnatal depletion isn't just about physiology—it's also about how and why mothers don't get the emotional and social support they need when they need it the most.

So I started reading about other cultures to see if there were any sociological clues that could point me in the right direction. Was postnatal depletion really unique to our Western culture? The more I read, the more I realized that many other cultures had stunning commonalities about how they managed their postpartum care. A depth of conscious practices, rituals, and ceremony—plus the support and respect for the recovery of mothers—has been embedded in different cultural fabrics all over the world since at least the start of recorded history. There was a standard of care given to mothers postpartum that has been lost to modern Western culture.

I think it can be helpful to take a look at the wisdom of some of these cultural practices and try to embrace as many of them as will fit into your life. Many of these traditions have a postpartum diet, in which the mother is given foods that are high in fat, nutrient dense, and easy to digest. Even better, someone else does the shopping and cooking! She has an army of helpers on hand to allow her to sleep and rest. She has these helpers showing her how to best do the hands-on baby care of feeding, changing, and bathing. She can relax in the knowledge that she is in a safe, nurturing place with those who only want the best for her and her new baby.

These cultures also share the notion of protected time—what is sometimes referred to as confinement but what really entails privacy, respect, and protection—with appropriate social support for the mother to fully recover after she gives birth. As a medical student I used to joke about one of the abbreviations found on the prenatal card that pregnant women would carry with them when attending visits with midwives or specialists. For the expected date of delivery (EDD) of the baby, there would usually be an EDC (estimated date of confinement). The medical students would tease one another that maybe pregnancy was like a prison sentence, and as ambitious students, we should remain childless lest we (horrors!) need to be confined ourselves.

This joke faded from my consciousness when a good friend of mine, who'd lived for thirty years in Ladakh, located in the Himalayan region of India, told me about the social support for newborns in traditional Ladakhi culture. There, when a baby was born, ten adults would be assigned to that baby to assist in various aspects of his or her initial and ongoing care through the child's entire upbringing. Imagine having that kind of support ingrained into our society!

Following is a sampling of traditions I have encountered from my years of research on birth practices. It will give you an appreciation of how complex the postnatal experience can be, and how diverse the cultural norms are, and perhaps you'll find something that resonates with you and can be adapted to your own modern life.

EXAMPLES OF POSTNATAL SUPPORT IN DIFFERENT CULTURES

China

In China, the practice of *zuo yue zi* literally means "sitting out the moon," or "the sitting month." This takes place right after the baby is born. Traditionally, the mother does not even leave the house—her only role is to breastfeed the baby, and her mother-in-law helps oversee the caretaking and does much of the food preparation and chores. This takes place over a four- or five-week period by keeping the mother warm, secluded, and rested—which is where the sitting out (resting) the moon (a month or lunar cycle) comes from.

The diet for the new mom during this month typically includes special types of chicken, soup, and large quantities of eggs and milk. Aside from the milk, raw and cold food is avoided. In Hong Kong, the Chinese also consider pig trotters served with ginger vinegar to be particularly nutritious for new moms, along with an herbal tea called *sheng hua tang*, said to promote energy and relieve exhaustion.

This system of lifestyle and dietary practices has been a central part of Chinese culture for at least a thousand years. The home was treated like a cocoon protected from visitors. I can only imagine the incredible opportunity for maternal-infant bonding that could take place under such a supportive system.

Korea

In Korea, *san-ho-jori* is a postpartum convention, still practiced in most traditional families, that typically lasts for twenty-one days following birth. The mother sleeps, eats, and nurses the baby during this time. She is encouraged to drink large amounts of hot tea as well as seaweed soup rich in calcium and iron, which are thought to assist in the production of breast milk. As in China, new moms are cautioned to avoid raw and cold foods.

India

In northern India, it is common to see the interesting practice of "mother roasting," in which the mother is kept warm for ten to forty days after the birth by a fire lit by the husband at the door of the house where the baby was born. The fire is kept going with special mustard and chaff; apart from keeping the mother warm, it is said to help keep *bhuts,* or demons, at bay. In the Punjab area, the mother is fed rich foods that are warming for the body and are often heavily laden with almonds and pistachios. In the coastal regions of southern India, a new mother is fed a special healing dish called a *marunta*, which consists of a fish called *kudipu meen* that is cooked with ginger, pepper, dill, and white garlic (nutritious and warming) and is eaten exclusively for the first twelve days.

Nepal

In traditional Nepalese culture, the new mother spends the first eleven days in a darkened and calm room with her baby. On the eleventh day she is welcomed out of the room for the baby's naming ceremony. She typically consumes a diet rich in high-energy foods, including ghee, hardened molasses, and caraway soup.

Tibet

There are no formal birth attendants or midwives in Tibetan culture. Instead, female relatives and the husband are on hand for the birth. Afterward, the new mom is given nourishing foods, including milk, meat stew, and bone broths. Salted butter tea is consumed regularly during the pregnancy and afterward, which helps give the baby nourishing fats through the mother's breast milk. For pregnant and nursing mothers, a sacred fortifying food consisting of small fish from Lake Manasarovar at the base of the sacred Mount Kailash is especially cherished.

Hmong / Southeast Asia

Hmong culture practices a thirty- to forty-day confinement called *nyob nruab hlis*. The mother is cared for by a single female relative in a separate part of the house with no contact with the outside world during this period. In the first three days, she sleeps on a straw-type bed by a fire. After three days, the bed is burned but the mother continues to stay by the fire. The first meal she has after the birth is a poached chicken egg with white pepper. In the following ten days she eats only hot rice and chicken soup imbued with greens and herbs. These greens, called *tshuaj qaib,* are considered very important for her recovery. Pork and fish may be included in the diet after ten days and boiled vegetables can be introduced after twenty days. No raw food is allowed.

The new mom is also not allowed to perform any duties for the first ten days and only light duties thereafter. She must avoid the cold and may not have sex for the entire confinement period.

Malawi

Traditional Malawian culture has a one-month confinement period during which the mother, to ensure she gets the best possible sleep, will sleep on a mat separate from her husband's. Only a few family members are allowed to hold the baby. After the confinement, the mother is allowed to bathe in a special herb bath. She then discards her confinement clothes. The child is not considered an individual for at least one month (often longer), at which time the baby is bathed in medicinal herbs and given its name.

Zimbabwe

Kusungira is practiced in traditional Zimbabwean culture. During her third trimester, the mother travels back to her parents' home and returns to her husband soon after the birth. She is put in isolation and is cared for by one female relative and the traditional birth assistant for one to three months while all household work and chores are done for her.

Aboriginal Australia

In traditional Australian culture, the term *aboriginal* is similar in meaning to the term *European*—it denotes a geographical area and not necessarily any cultural similarity between aboriginal tribes. In fact, aboriginal culture is extremely diverse and varied, much like the Native American culture in North America is.

One deeply significant practice that is universal among aboriginal cultures is the smoking ceremony, which is designed to strengthen both mother and child and to help stimulate the production of breast milk. A hole is dug in the ground and a fire is prepared with a special type of wood. Pieces of red ant pit or nest are added to the fire. Once the fire has died down and the red ant pit has turned to ash, the mother, holding the baby wrapped in a blanket, squats over the hole. Once she starts getting very hot, she urinates over the ash, allowing herself and the baby to be embraced by the steam. The mother then spends another fifteen to twenty minutes squatting over the hole without her baby. This is a night ceremony and typically occurs consecutively over three to four nights.

Native Americans

The most common practice is that of the "lying-in time," whereby women attend to the new mother and baby, pampering the mother with special nourishment, grooming, washing, steaming in a sweat lodge, and massage. The Shawnee Indians require ten days of lying-in; for the Picuris Pueblo Indians it is thirty days. The Hopi purification ritual requires a twenty-day lying-in, during which time the mother is not allowed to have the sun shine on her. On the night of the nineteenth day, a great feast is prepared and the baby is rubbed in ash. The father announces the arrival of the sun at dawn. When the sun's rays touch the baby's face for the first time, the grandmother of the tribe chooses the baby's name. The mother then goes to the sweat lodge to complete her purification. And in the San Juan Paiute tradition, the mother and husband must both observe certain prohibitions for the first thirty days, which include not eating any form of meat and avoiding salt and cold water. They may touch their hair and face with only a scratching stick and not their hands. When the thirty days have passed, the parents bathe in cold water, trim the ends of their hair, and paint their faces with red ocher.

DO YOU HAVE POSTNATAL DEPLETION?

My life goal is to enable all mothers to have access to information that will help them not only prevent depletion but also recover from it. The bottom line is that if you want a healthy society, you need to have healthy communities. To have healthy communities, you have to start with a healthy family. If you want a healthy family, you need to have the mother in the best possible health physically, emotionally, mentally, and spiritually. I want to help you close the doors to postnatal depletion one at a time, and the first step is understanding how postnatal depletion is impacting your life.

Following is a questionnaire designed to help you identify the symptoms in your life that might be pointing toward postnatal depletion. I hope that you find this informative and helpful; with the right help, it's possible to resolve these symptoms and begin to reclaim yourself!

	No 0	Sometimes 1	Frequently 2	All the time 3
Have you had a medical condition start during or after pregnancy?				
Do you feel you have digestive issues that have worsened since the birth of your child? These issues may include constipation/diarrhea, flatulence/ abdominal pain, and/or lethargy associated with meals.				
Do you experience severe fatigue?				
Do you feel exhausted on waking?				
Do you fall asleep unintentionally when putting the children to bed?				
Do you have sensitivity to bright light (or repetitive sounds) and are you easily startled?				
Are you experiencing levels of anxiety that are way above your norm?				
Do you feel you are a "light sleeper" and are overly aware while you're sleeping?				
Do you have any sex drive or a healthy libido?				
Do you experience severe brain fog?				
Are you struggling to keep up with basic self-care, such as showering, grooming, and preparing meals for yourself?				
Are you experiencing a significant loss of confidence and self-esteem?				
Do you have a sense of isolation and lack of support?				

	No 0	Sometimes 1	Frequently 2	All the time 3
Do you feel that "there is *no* time for me"?				
Do you feel overwhelmed and unable to cope?				
Do you feel a sense of guilt/shame or failure around your role as a mother?				

Score 20 or more: Postnatal depletion very likely

Score 15 to 19: Postnatal depletion likely

Score below 15: Postnatal depletion unlikely

CHAPTER 2

Physical Symptoms and Why They Worsen

As you know, pregnancy takes an enormous toll on your body. While you're watching your belly grow on the outside, on the inside your body is undergoing incredible changes and stresses to give the developing fetus the best care possible. You've likely endured morning sickness, energy that flags, food cravings, hair that is thick and shiny one day and falling out the next, skin that glows or that might suddenly develop acne, and swollen ankles. Or maybe you've been lucky and sailed through, feeling better and more joyful than you've ever felt before.

Whatever your pregnancy symptoms, and whether you feel the effects of pregnancy's physical stress or not, your body is getting depleted because the developing fetus needs so many nutrients. So let's take a look in this chapter at how *physical* depletion happens and what some of the most common symptoms of it are. (I'll discuss emotional depletion symptoms, like anxiety and baby brain, in the next chapter.)

THE START OF PHYSICAL POSTNATAL DEPLETION

The placenta is one of the most amazing structures in the human body. Without it, no fetus could ever survive. But the placenta also triggers the physical symptoms of postnatal depletion.

The word *placenta* comes from the Greek, meaning "plate" or "discoid." This is because the placenta actually does look like a dinner plate

THE PHYSICAL SYMPTOMS OF POSTNATAL DEPLETION

These are the most common physical symptoms of postnatal depletion. If you are depleted, it is absolutely normal to have one or all of them:

- Baby brain
- Fatigue, often debilitating
- Insomnia or disturbed/nonrestful sleep
- Loss of skin elasticity, skin dryness, softer nails, thinning hair, increased translucency of the teeth, receding gums, easier bruising
- Sensitivity to light and sound

or disc attached to the side of the uterus, with the umbilical cord going to the baby. After conception, a newly forming fetus will focus all its efforts on establishing a healthy placenta.

What the Placenta Does

The placenta has several important roles. It has a very complex and unique function as a corridor of information from the mother to the fetus and then back to the mother:

- It acts as a filter, via the umbilical cord, allowing in from the mother all the good stuff required for proper development, while preventing toxins from reaching the fetus.
- It functions as a sensor, determining what the fetus needs and regulating the absorption of everything from amino acids to vitamins, fats, and oxygen.
- It operates as a hormone factory, producing high levels of estrogen, progesterone, and cortisol, to name a few, for both the baby and the mother.

What's also interesting is that the placenta and the fetal hypothalamus both develop at the same time. The hypothalamus is a crucial hormone-producing gland within the brain. Many hormones produced by the placenta share structural similarities with hormones produced by the mother's brain. In other words, the mother's brain starts to become influenced by the fetal placenta. This starts the "software upgrade" that begins the initiation into motherhood.

In other words, these placental hormones actually *start to change the wiring of a mother's brain* so that she is more interested in, more sensitive to, and more aware of the needs of her growing baby. The motto to remember is "If the fetus requires, the mother obliges."

Though there's not much research, it appears that the smell and taste centers in the brains of pregnant mothers get extra wiring; this could, to a large extent, account for the nausea associated with early pregnancy as well as the unusual food cravings that pregnancy is renowned for. The emotional centers also get a big upgrade, with emotional reasoning, intelligence, and sensitivity all being affected. While these changes are useful in helping you bond with and be able to read the subtle and not-so-subtle cues of your newborn more deeply, they can also be a bit confusing for mothers who may not be aware that they might happen or be prepared when they do.

The Placental Lining

The lining of the placenta is unique, one of the most intriguing organs ever created. It has millions upon millions of finger-like projections (called chorionic villi, in case you're interested) that reach into the lining of the uterus. These villi are lined with a cell type known as syncytiotrophoblasts, which are similar in appearance to plastic wrap. A syncytiotrophoblast is one cell layer thick with no dividing cell wall and is essentially a single cell with thousands of nuclei. Not only does it line the placenta; it also encapsulates the whole baby. Think of it as a balloon that marks off where the baby stops and the mother starts.

As part of the placental system, the uterus is designed to leak the mother's blood into the space between the lining of the uterus and the syncytiotrophoblastic balloon around the fetus. This is called the intervillous space. The fetus needs this blood to be there, because this is how the fetus gets its nourishment.

The Importance of Your Type of Placenta

In nature there are two types of placentas. Most mammals have a placenta that looks like two hands with interlaced fingers, one hand being the mother and one hand being the baby. Humans, along with great apes, have a different, more ancient type, called a hemochorial-type placenta, which looks more like a hand grabbing a clenched fist or a head of broccoli. The advantage to humans of this type of placenta is that its incredibly high surface area allows for the increase of nutrients and fats that pass from mother to baby in the last trimester. The downside to this type of placenta is that when the mother has inflammation or an infection, it can be harder to contain and prevent from spreading to the baby. This is one of the reasons for the adverse outcomes of pregnancy, such as preeclampsia.

Before you ask yourself why this is relevant, let me explain. The human placenta is much more invasive than any other placenta found in nature, as it extends farther and deeper into the lining of the uterus. This has to do with the incredible nutrient and energy load that a human fetus requires. Growing and fueling a new human brain requires a lot of resources. In fact, 60 percent of the total nutrients allocated by the mother for pregnancy are directed to the development of her fetus's brain. (This number is closer to only 20 percent in other mammals.) In addition, up to 7 grams of fat is required to be transferred across the placental interface every day in the latter stages of pregnancy. No other animal comes close to this.

Why is this important to know? Because we've evolved to become who we are as a result of our disproportionately large brains. Because the brain is made up of various fats—which is why a low-fat diet will never be good for your brain!—it is essential for our survival to have an effective way of delivering fat to the developing fetus.

So what does all this information have to do with postnatal depletion? Well, the only way we can get 7 grams of fat across the placental interface and to the fetus every day is for the placental lining to have a huge surface area. This has a very real downside. This placental interface is more likely to have microhemorrhages, which are like tiny tears through the lining of the syncytiotrophoblastic balloon. The result? A leaky placenta that can cause and contribute to many of the problems seen during pregnancy and postnatally. Preeclampsia is just one of the life-threatening pregnancy complications that scientists know is caused by placental leaking, but they don't yet know how significant these leaks can be for other conditions. Evidence points to leaks as contributing to the development of autoimmune diseases in the mother during and after pregnancy.

This link is an essential piece of the puzzle in our understanding of how, why, and where postnatal depletion begins. And from what we are beginning to understand about the integrity of the placental lining, it all has to do with *inflammation*.

THE ROLE OF INFLAMMATION IN POSTNATAL DEPLETION

A normal pregnancy is characterized by mild systemic inflammation. It is low-grade and it is controlled by the complex interplay between the mother and the fetus. It is part of what happens when a woman is growing a baby inside her. People often think of inflammation as the redness, heat, and swelling that might accompany an infection or injury that your body is fighting off or trying to heal, but there are actually different types of inflammation. With pregnancy, inflammation is actually a healthy and normal part of the process.

Think of it this way: if your body is likened to a large city, each home is a cell in your body; the roads are the blood vessels; and the organs are the different districts, such as industrial, financial, and residential, and so on. Inflammation is like the earth-moving equipment, power tools, lawn mowers, and plows that the city government keeps on hand for maintenance and cleaning up after a snowstorm—and also to take care of new projects like making a baby!

Sometimes, in this city, buildings have to be removed to make way for a new development. The destructive part of this (and to a lesser extent the constructive part) is inflammation. The city workers (or the enzymes within and without the cells) receive a permit, telling them where to go and what to do; in your body, these permits or messages are called cytokines. The cytokines allow for the construction, repair, and rebuilding teams to bring in their equipment and start working. This mild inflammation prepares your body for pregnancy and delivery in all kinds of ways. It allows your immune system to react properly and not reject the baby; it allows the ligaments in your pelvis to soften slightly in preparation for a vaginal delivery; it allows for breast tissue development so that you're ready to breastfeed as soon as the baby is born; and it allows for the increase of blood vessels to the placenta and the allocation of nutrients to the baby.

Things get into trouble, however, if there are too few or too many of these inflammatory cytokines. If there is not enough inflammation, the placenta will not grow properly and miscarriage is more likely. But too much inflammation can contribute to complications of pregnancy such as reduced fetal growth, premature labor, and preeclampsia. And if a mother is already dealing with inflammation caused by a gut problem, poor diet, hormone imbalance, or other medical issues, the extra inflammation caused by pregnancy can further derail and compromise her ability to contain and deal with it. This causes even more bodily stress and depleted nutrients, and it paves the way for the common symptoms of postnatal depletion.

COMMON INFLAMMATION DIAGNOSES

- Hashimoto's disease and other autoimmune diseases, such as lupus and rheumatoid arthritis
- Postpartum thyroiditis
- Inhalant allergies, such as atopic hay fever and asthma
- Irritable bowel syndrome

THE ROLE OF AUTOIMMUNE DISORDERS IN POSTNATAL DEPLETION

There is another potential trigger for postnatal depletion, and that is an autoimmune disorder or disease.

Your immune system is constantly neutralizing and clearing out foreign material that it perceives as dangerous or attacking. Normally, this is a good thing; if flu virus antigens have entered your body because an infected person sneezed on you, you want your body to invade and destroy them as quickly as possible.

If, however, a small amount of foreign material from the fetus passes into the mother, you can develop an autoimmune disorder. When this happens, your cells mistakenly attack one another, and if not dealt with, an autoimmune disorder can lead to progressive damage to that part of the body. The disorder may be mild or it can be severe, making mothers very sick.

Having an autoimmune disorder doesn't automatically result in postnatal depletion, but I do see these disorders often in my patients who *are* depleted. And even if the autoimmune disorder wasn't the cause of postnatal depletion, the disorder can certainly make it a whole lot worse.

COMMON AUTOIMMUNE DISORDERS

Hashimoto's disease—thyroid inflammation that can lead to hypothyroidism, causing the body to become even more sluggish and lethargic.

Inflammatory bowel disease—digestive tract inflammation that interferes with the body's ability to absorb the nutrients it needs, such as vitamin B_{12} and calcium.

CHANGES TO YOUR POSTNATAL BODY

In the first six weeks after your baby is born, you may experience numerous common conditions and symptoms, including hemorrhoids, increased sweating, urinary incontinence, constipation, hair loss, back pain, breast changes, and vaginal changes (including pain and discharge as the uterus contracts and heals). Your abdomen can take some time to reduce in size, leaving most mothers with a belly bulge. All these typically improve, if not within the first six weeks, then over several months.

What is rarely talked about are the common long-term changes to a woman's body following delivery. There is even a lot of confusion about which changes can be attributed simply to aging and which are pregnancy related. Unfortunately, there just hasn't been enough research on these issues to provide definitive answers. But here are some things we do know.

Breast Size

It is normal for breasts to get significantly bigger before and after birth and with breastfeeding. After breastfeeding is finished, it is not uncommon for there to continue to be a release of a small amount of milk, what looks like colostrum, for many months.

What is particularly distressing for many mothers is that breast size, after breast feeding, can often be smaller than it was prepregnancy, and the more children you breastfeed, the saggier the breasts will be. This is related not to the physical act of breastfeeding, surprisingly enough, but to the action of the hormones of breastfeeding and the reduced stimulatory effect of progesterone and estrogen on the breast tissue after breastfeeding.

Belly Bulge

It takes about six weeks for the uterus to fully contract to its normal size, but due to the stretching of the skin and the laxity of both the abdominal wall and the pelvic floor, the bulge can remain ever after. Diastasis recti, or a separation of the abdominal muscles, can occur in up to 60 percent of pregnancies. It happens because the connecting tissues get thinner as a mother's belly expands and bulges farther forward during pregnancy. This can often slowly resolve, but 30 percent of women can still have this one *year* after the birth of their baby! Some of my mothers have described it as a kangaroo pouch.

Feet

It is not uncommon for mothers to need larger shoes—up to an extra half inch—after pregnancy. The American College of Obstetrics and Gynecologists recommends that average-size women gain between twenty-five and thirty-five pounds during pregnancy. This puts extra weight on the arches of your feet and, combined with the hormone relaxin, which relaxes ligaments not only in the pelvis but sometimes also in the arches of the feet, causes a slight flattening of the arch.

Hair

During pregnancy, high estrogen levels prolong your hair's growing phase, causing less hair than usual to fall out. After you give birth, your estrogen levels plummet, and you begin to shed more hair, sometimes in alarming amounts. It can take about six to twelve months for the rate of new growth and shedding to return to what it once was.

Menstruation

After the uterus stretches during pregnancy, it can be left with up to twice as much surface area as it had in prepregnancy, so it is common for menstrual cycles to be heavier after a pregnancy.

Skin

Skin issues during pregnancy, such as suddenly getting acne or seeing preexisting acne disappear, are common. One of the first changes many women notice during pregnancy is the darkening of their nipples. Melanin, the hormone responsible for the pigmentation of your skin, increases during pregnancy, so this can affect not only your nipples but other parts of your skin as well. It is also common to see melasma, darkened patches of skin on your lips, nose, cheeks, and/or forehead. Other areas that may darken are scars, freckles, moles, labia, and the skin under your armpits. Stretch marks of pregnancy will also darken, as will the midline running from the belly button to the pubic bone. These pigmented areas usually fade with time postbirth.

BABY BRAIN

Have you found that you're sometimes in a stupor, and time seems to go by in a flash? That tasks you once did in a few seconds are now taking minutes? That you can't remember where you put the baby's bottle and you find it in the freezer, along with your keys, a few hours later? That you forgot what was in the article about baby food that you were just reading?

No, you're not going crazy or losing your mind. You just have preghead, Momnesia, or what most of my patients call baby brain!

There is no scientific consensus on what baby brain is, and research on the topic is extremely limited. But every single new mom who's experienced this debilitating mental fog knows exactly what I'm talking about. They don't care why they have it—they just want to know when it's going away. If you're interested in understanding what's actually happening, though, read on.

Baby Brain Cause 1: Your Brain Is Getting Reprogrammed for Baby

Baby brain is the result of a unique set of events. It is most likely due to the reprogramming of the mother's brain, triggered by the placenta, to ensure that a deep sense of bonding with the baby occurs. Part of this reprogramming includes increased numbers of neurons and neuronal connections in the taste and smell centers of a mother's brain. There are also increased neuronal connections and extra neutrons installed in the emotional centers of the mother's brain, including the amygdala, which increases the mother's emotional intelligence. (IQ might also increase slightly, although a lot more research needs to be done on this topic.)

So what happens to a mother's brain when she's pregnant? There are enormously elevated levels of the female hormone progesterone, which is involved in the maturation of the new neuron connections just described. This also tends to have a pleasantly sedating effect on the mother's brain. There are also increased levels of estrogen, the other female hormone, which seems to be involved in helping the proliferation of new neurons in the brain as well. These elevated levels of progesterone and estrogen together protect the mother against the "neuro-stress" of high cortisol, the hormone released when your body perceives any kind of stress. (For more on cortisol, see the section "Baby Brain Cause 4: The Stress Response" on page 35.) In other words, these changes in hormones and brain wiring are intended to make a mother hypervigilant to protect the developing fetus (which is good) but not necessarily anxious or in a state of hyperarousal (which can be unnecessarily stressful).

These specific pregnancy-brain upgrades, with increased neural connections within the mother's brain, are what psychologists refer to as being learning ready. In other words, the brain is primed to be a better learner on all topics. In fact, even though there is some disagreement about this in the scientific community, it seems that cognition significantly improves during pregnancy. Moms-to-be become smarter. You knew that already, of course!

All of your senses can be heightened as well. The part of your brain involved in emotional skills becomes more active, making it better able to process facial emotions—presumably to help with baby bonding. An enhanced sense of smell makes you more discerning with food and able to lock in with that delicious new baby smell when your baby is born. This in part accounts for the strange cravings that pregnant moms often have, as well as the random aversions to foods that they used to love. These aversions can be particularly strong around spoiled or new foods as a precaution to protect the fetus, although this subtle tuning can certainly seem random when you want a mustard sandwich at 3:00 a.m.!

As this is happening, your brain shrinks slightly during the last trimester of pregnancy. It's nothing to worry about as it's temporary; your brain will go back to normal by the time your baby is about six months old. This is pertinent for baby brain, though, because your brain doesn't shrink all over—it's more like getting restructured so that some sections of it become larger and other sections become smaller. It seems that the taste and smell centers plus the emotional hub (the amygdala) are the main beneficiaries.

Researchers aren't quite sure why this happens, but what it does show is that the imminent arrival of the baby will literally change the hard-wiring of your brain in preparation for his or her arrival into this world.

So if you've been struggling to figure out why you're having a hard time thinking, you aren't going crazy. Baby brain is the result of your mental-processing rate's being automatically slowed down to enable you to become more attentive and able to instantly read the subtle cues coming from your baby so that you are better able to bond and attend to your infant's needs. I also believe that your ability to multitask, especially if you're trying to do things quickly, gets very adversely affected. Mothers I've worked with have said, "I don't have baby brain; I just wasn't listening to you," because they feel like they have a list of things to take care of simmering on the back burner at all times.

Tasks involving time awareness (e.g., planning out your day efficiently) and project management (e.g., trying to organize a kid's birthday party) may seem unusually difficult or take a lot more time than expected; multitasking at your desk, which was once easy, is now impossible. This can be extremely frustrating, especially because the list of things you need to manage is getting longer and the time you have in which you need to get everything done feels shorter than ever. You might find this astonishing, but you're actually becoming slightly *smarter*—but with a skill set that is leading you to have slower but more insightful thinking and sensory enhancement. While these changes in brain function are critical to your role as a new mother, they can also disrupt what were once your regular thought processes.

Baby Brain Cause 2: Sleep Deprivation

I'll bet you look back at your late teens and twenties and marvel at how easy it once was to go out all night partying with your friends or pull all-nighters studying for exams and then be able to go to work or classes the next day, tired and yawning but still able to function. When mothers are younger, it's easier for their bodies to handle the demands of regular round-the-clock feedings. For older moms in their thirties and forties, however, the once-innate resilience to sleep disturbance decreases, and it becomes harder for them to cope with the effects of broken or reduced sleep. And as you likely know, lack of sleep is no joke.

There are some complex and wonderful things that occur during sleep to help replenish your brain and body. The brain does a lot of its housekeeping, including clearing toxins and repairing damaged cells, during sleep. It also performs a recalibration of your senses, a bit like adjusting the colors and brightness of a computer screen. This occurs only during sleep, as does the production of restorative hormones, such as growth hormone and DHEA (dehydroepiandrosterone). The liver does most of its detoxification work and the gut does most of its digestion work while you're asleep, and these energy-intensive processes work better and more efficiently when sleep comes in one consolidated block.

When you don't get enough sleep, particularly if you are awakened during the deepest sleep when your body and brain are trying to replenish themselves, you feel terrible. It can have profound effects on all your motor functions, your mental functions, and your mood (which I'll discuss in both chapters 3 and 8).

Getting enough sleep is a really big deal. Chronic sleep deprivation increases day-to-day negative emotions, such as sadness, anger, and negative self-talk, leaving you at higher risk for depression. It can also reduce self-esteem and marital satisfaction. That's why it's particularly devastating that pregnancy and parenthood can disrupt your sleep patterns just when you need them the most. For a more detailed discussion, see chapter 8.

This is what can happen when you're facing sleep deprivation:

- You have trouble finding the right words: "Can you pass me the… thingy?"
- You can't multitask in the way that you used to: "Has the washing machine finished its cycle? Oh, wait, I've got to go pee, but I think I'm hungry so I need to make a sandwich. Do I have to go to the post office today or tomorrow?"
- You struggle more with decision-making tasks, such as comparing and selecting insurance policies or determining which cleaning products

are best to use. Making decisions about your day-to-day life can lead to instant overwhelm.

- Your alertness and reaction times are adversely affected. Your reflexes slow down. You are more accident-prone. Many studies have shown that chronic sleep deprivation has an effect on alertness and reaction times equivalent to a 0.05 to 0.1 percent blood alcohol content (BAC). (In the United States a driver is considered legally impaired with a BAC of 0.08 percent.)
- You have a harder time dealing with cravings. Because your hormone levels decrease when you're sleep deprived, you can develop resistance to hormones such as insulin and leptin. Insulin is made by the pancreas in response to spikes of blood sugar after you eat carbohydrates or any food with sugars in it. Leptin, produced by fat cells, essentially informs the brain about the overall fat stores in your body. If your body stops responding to these hormones, it can throw your blood sugar and appetite out of whack, leading to increased cravings for junk food and sugar. Good sleep actually helps reduce food cravings!
- Your immune system is weakened, making it harder to fight off infections, such as the common cold or flu.

Baby Brain Cause 3: Nutrient Robbery

Let's go back to the placenta again. The miracle of growing a baby inside you comes at the expense of many of the nutrients that *you* need. That placenta is going to grab what it can, even if your own levels are low. That robbery of nutrients and reserves in service of creating and birthing a baby contributes to baby brain and the depletion that mothers experience during pregnancy and after the birth.

One of the biggest nutrient grabs is that of omega-3 fatty acids, which you probably know about if you take fish oil supplements. A developing fetus has a particular need for the important omega-3 fatty acid DHA (docosahexaenoic acid), which is essential for the healthy development of the brain, eyes, and central nervous system. The only place to get it is from the Mommy DHA Reservoir, located in the mother's brain. (Did you know that one-third of the dry weight of the brain is made of DHA? Now you do!) I think this is why so many prenatal vitamins make a point to advertise their DHA content and include it as standard, but the dosages are often insufficient.

I believe, although I have yet to find any science to back me up on this, that it is as if the mother is giving tiny amounts of her own brain to ensure that the baby can make his or her own. What an amazing example of altruism! But moms-to-be pay the price for this selfless act. DHA is an integral part of the coating that surrounds and protects the neurons in the brain. Without enough of it, you can expect to experience a downgrade in mental functioning and an upswing in overthinking and anxiety. Extra DHA supplements are an essential way to help speed up the recovery from postnatal depletion. (I'll discuss how to replace these "stolen" nutrients in chapters 4 and 5.)

Baby Brain Cause 4: The Stress Response

We are evolutionarily designed for periods of hardworking, high physical demands followed by rest and relaxation—stress on/stress off. All hunter-gatherer tribes spend more time relaxing and socializing than they do hunting and gathering. This back-and-forth dynamic between stress and relaxation helps trigger and maintain healthy levels of cellular repair, hormone production, and liver detoxification; it also supports ideal immune and digestive function.

What we are not designed for, yet what's become an almost default position of the Western way of being, is stress on/stress *on*. In this dynamic, the stress button is never switched off. Your body doesn't reset itself back to normal. Instead, it is bathed in stress hormones until you're completely wiped out. All the bodily functions described previously become compromised, leading to more and more fatigue until you feel completely wiped out. Dr. Libby Weaver describes this wonderfully in her book *Rushing Woman's Syndrome*. It is an essential read for my highly stressed mothers.

As a reaction to this ongoing and constant stress, the body goes from overproducing to underproducing cortisol, resulting in a deficit of this important hormone. Among its many jobs, cortisol regulates circadian rhythm (our sense of day and night), energy utilization, and that feeling of consistent energy that takes us through the day.

Cortisol is somctimcs called the challenge hormone. It's your body's drill sergeant. It gets you up in the morning, and then it winds you down so you're able to get to sleep. But when your drill sergeant was up all night in the trenches (which is how you can feel when your baby is screaming and you're desperate to get back to sleep!), the last thing it wants to do is get up out of a comfy bed in the morning. Your drill sergeant is going to be either awfully mad and yelling or sluggish, slow, and cranky. Which is you with baby brain, feeling totally burned-out.

Another one of cortisol's important functions is to work in combination with your thyroid gland to regulate how your cells use their energy. The thyroid secretes hormones that are responsible for regulating your metabolism. Your body produces T4 (thyroxine), an inactive hormone, which is then activated to T3 (triiodothyronine), a form of the hormone your body can actually use. When your thyroid hormones are checked via a blood test, T3 and T4 are always measured. The amount of free T3 (in ratio to reverse T3) determines how well your thyroid is actually functioning.

I am growing increasingly concerned about the prevalence of thyroid issues, because I see them affecting more and more younger women, especially when they become pregnant. When I was a medical student in the early 1990s, I typically saw thyroid issues only in my postmenopausal seniors. Fast-forward a few years, and I started seeing thyroid issues occurring more commonly in middle-age women. In more recent years, my patients with both underperforming and overperforming thyroids are even younger and often present with autoimmune thyroid disorders such as Hashimoto's disease. I'm convinced that there's something about the modern lifestyle contributing to this thyroid phenomenon.

During pregnancy, some women will have a reduced thyroid reserve. This means their thyroid is less able to increase its hormone production when it's most needed. When you're pregnant, your T4 and T3 production should increase by 50 percent to meet the requirements for you and your developing fetus. When there's a crisis going on—such as an extra stressor like baby-induced sleep deprivation—the thyroid can get stingy. This is the same evolutionary mechanism that got humans through famine, drought, and other life-threatening stresses—but I don't think that's much of a consolation to you when you're too tired to function properly! One saving grace is that the fetus is very much protected from the storm and won't be affected unless the situation is severe.

With thyroid problems becoming more prevalent in younger women, it is also becoming more common for women to require thyroid replacement during pregnancy—and after. Nearly one in six Australian women have thyroid problems after the baby is born, and they have a 50 percent chance of developing a hypothyroid condition in the ensuing seven years.

That is a shocking figure. If your thyroid is underfunctioning, you can suffer from chronic lethargy. You are not going to want to get out of bed because you literally do not have any energy to spare.

SENSITIVITY TO LIGHT AND SOUND

Have you ever noticed that a stressed or angry person will often have small or even pinpoint pupils? The more relaxed someone is, the bigger their pupils. This is the result of the balance between the sympathetic nervous system (which activates the fight/flight or freeze response) and the parasympathetic nervous symptom (which regulates rest and digestion); together they make up our ancient regulating system, the autonomic nervous system. The autonomic (or automatic, if you like) nervous system performs all the bodily tasks that we take for granted, like breathing, heart pumping, and digestion. It also primes the body for any perceived threats.

Your brain requires an incredible amount of energy to maintain a state of hyperalertness. What regulates the availability of this energy is cortisol and, to a lesser extent, adrenaline (or epinephrine). As discussed earlier, if your cortisol level is low, your body struggles to remain alert and attentive.

One of the medical tests we can do to assess for low cortisol is called the iris contraction test. In a darkened room, a beam of light from a small flashlight is shone from the side of the head toward your pupil. If your adrenal function is normal, your iris should remain contracted with the pupil remaining small for up to two minutes. If you are depleted, however, with a low-adrenal state, your eye may be able to remain contracted for only ten to fifteen *seconds* before the pupil starts to dilate and then constrict again—almost like it is pulsating. This explains why, if you have cortisol depletion, you might find it so hard to go out in the bright sunshine, why any harsh lighting automatically makes you feel awful, and why you can't leave the house without strong, dark sunglasses.

A similar phenomenon occurs with a depleted mother's hearing. Sounds seem to be amplified, and combined with the sensory enhancement discussed earlier in this chapter, this can lead to a very short fuse that all parents know only too well. What we see with postnatal depletion is an accumulation of issues over time in which the physical symptoms of fatigue, difficulty with concentration, and overwhelming anxiety start to build on one another in a gradual and sometimes not-so-gradual way. Over time, this begins to take its toll.

Until I started studying postnatal depletion, I was always a little surprised when mothers reported that they were adversely sensitive to the noise of their children. But understanding cortisol's role in this made me realize that these kids aren't being too noisy (kids are noisy by nature!); rather, their mothers find it hard to cope with and filter out the noise. Perhaps this is how the saying "Children should be seen and not heard" originated.

Once your depletion has been corrected, you'll be able to stash the sunglasses and stop shushing the kids when they're running around. But in the meantime, know that there's nothing wrong with you as a parent if you're having a hard time being around your kids and their boisterous, loud playtime.

CHAPTER 3

Emotional Symptoms and Why They Worsen

Why do so many moms feel so bad after their beloved babies are born? Or rather, why do so many moms feel so bad *emotionally* even when they're thrilled and delighted with their new babies?

This happened to my patient Candace. "You know what's weird?" she said, her eyes filling with tears as she looked down at the beautiful little baby asleep in her lap. "I feel everything so intensely all the time, but it still feels like my brain had stopped. Like I can see all these bright colors of joy and sadness, and then I just get numb. And apathetic. Like this fog is still there even when I'm incredibly content to be a mother." She sighed. "I'm really worried because I'm starting to feel bad more often than I'm feeling good. I'm really irritable and I lose my temper." She started crying in earnest. "I'm even shouting at my kids when they're being angels, and at my husband, too. I love them so much. Why is this happening to me?"

"Well," I said. "A lot of the mothers who come to see me use the term *Groundhog Day*."

Candace laughed. "You got it. Yeah, it really feels like a merry-go-round that you can't get off," she added. "Sometimes if I have to think about cooking another meal or seeing another pile of dirty laundry, I feel like I could burst." Tears welled up in her eyes. "Then I just cry, feel like a failure, and get on with my day. I should be so happy I have everything that I need. I see the other moms and they seem to be keeping it together, and then I feel like I'm doing okay, but then the kids are fighting or my three-year-old doesn't want to wear that dress and I crack. When I haven't fallen asleep trying to read to the kids at bedtime, I just lie awake thinking and thinking. I don't necessarily want my old life back, but I used to do competitive sports, I used to love solving puzzles...I used to *do* things!"

I cannot count the number of women who come to me with stories like Candace's. When there is a new baby, the everyday logistics of feeding, dressing, cleaning, keeping everyone safe, and never mind being on time are and can be incredibly overwhelming. And when combined with all the physical aspects of postnatal depletion, the result can be profound and negative.

EMOTIONAL SYMPTOMS: THE DIRECT CAUSES AND EFFECTS

Causes:

- Physical changes to the mother's brain
- Hormonal changes
- Loss of sleep and disrupted circadian rhythm
- Change of role and confusion over new role vs. old role
- Reduced support, whether from work, society, family, or partner
- Poor preparation for the postdelivery role of being a new parent
- Social pressure, which can make struggling new moms feel like a failure

Effects:

- Anxiety
- Decreased libido
- Guilt/shame
- Inability to cope
- Loss of self-confidence
- Sense of isolation
- Sense of powerlessness/diminishment

I have heard a mother describe these feelings as the "worry train": sometimes there are very specific and unrelenting worries, such as the baby's health or the lack of a routine, but other times there are no precise fears—just a pervasive sense of vulnerability and that something bad could or might happen.

Anxiety can intensify after the birth of a first child; with a new baby comes uncertainty and the growing awareness of the enormity of the learning curve that the mother is on. Some women also harbor inappropriate expectations that everything will be perfect; these can stem from not having had prior experience with raising children coupled with an attachment to a former life where they enjoyed a feeling of being in control. It is a fraught time when idealism and realism collide.

Anxiety is an emotion. We have an emotion first, before we have a thought. We feel before we think. When the emotions are very strong, they can derail our thinking. Trying to outthink your emotions even when they are not highly charged is challenging, and we are not designed to be in state of high emotion for extended periods. Our emotional being should be like a strong tree that will sway with the winds of situational emotions but always return to the center. When we lose resilience, we can easily become overwhelmed, like a drooping tree, and may even develop a sense of resignation that things are never going to improve. I often see this in my postnatal patients. In a state of postnatal depletion, a whirlwind of unexpected feelings occurs. This in turn can enhance the emotional experience of postnatal depletion.

THE EMOTIONAL SYMPTOMS OF POSTNATAL DEPLETION

There are basically eight major emotions that emerge in the postnatal period:

- FEAR commonly manifests as anxiety, an inability to cope, procrastination and/or indecisiveness, and a sense of being easily overwhelmed.

- ANGER can fluctuate and is often internally targeted; it later manifests as guilt and shame.
- SADNESS, while similar to depression, is tinged with a sense of grief.
- JOY, a feeling of intense happiness, can be powerfully moving but can fluctuate like a yo yo, as many mothers know.
- DISGUST, usually internally targeted as self-hate or self-loathing, stems from feelings of inadequacy.
- LOSS OF TRUST can manifest both in one's own abilities and in the support that one, as a mother, is receiving.
- ANTICIPATION is a forward-looking emotion that can manifest in either a positive or a negative way, depending on whether that which is being looked forward to is regarded with pleasure or with worry.
- SURPRISE is a startle response that can be positive or negative.

If you find yourself experiencing any, most, or all of these emotions after the birth of your baby, you are not alone.

Before I go into the reasons why these negative feelings can arise, let's take a look at the difference between postnatal depletion (very common) and postpartum depression (less common).

POSTNATAL DEPLETION OR POSTPARTUM DEPRESSION?

The phenomenon of "baby blues"—a set of emotional symptoms that typically occur together and include a sense of distress, irritability, sensitivity, fluctuations in mood, and typically feeling very teary—occurs in up to 80 percent of new mothers. It usually begins about three days after the birth and can last up to two weeks.

Baby blues are the result of a big hormonal change in which women experience an immediate drop in progesterone, estrogen, and the stress hormone cortisol coupled with an immediate increase in prolactin (the hormone of lactation) and then a later rise in cortisol. For many moms, this hormonal situation passes quickly as the feel-good hormone oxytocin, as well as dopamine, the reward/pleasure brain neurotransmitter, is released in abundant amounts.

However, the precise sequence of hormone and brain-chemical fluctuations can be easily upset, which contributes to the negative emotions a mother may experience postnatally. For some mothers, the chemical balance doesn't shift back right away. Within the first twelve months of birth, the postpartum depression rate in Australia is approximately 13 percent; that's about one out of every eight Australian moms. The rate in the United States is 10 to 20 percent.

POSSIBLE FACTORS CONTRIBUTING TO DEPRESSION

Postpartum depression is caused by many different factors, and hormones tend to be the "amplifier," though not necessarily the cause.

- Genetic predisposition
- Past history of anxiety
- Difficulties during the pregnancy and/or delivery
- Relationship stress
- Lack of social support
- Worries about money

When under stress, the brain chemicals, or neurotransmitters, get out of whack, leading to fewer of the feel-good neurotransmitters (mostly serotonin) being released. Serotonin is needed to regulate brain functions like appetite, sleep, memory, and mood. Meanwhile, levels of melatonin, the hormone that supports both sleep and reproductive cycles, also decrease. Lack of sleep has a snowballing effect and can perpetuate the further progression of anxiety, sadness, and lethargy, which can be a part of depression. Is it any wonder that these sufferers feel terrible and have trouble sleeping?

Doctors who treat postpartum depression usually divide it into two types: nonmelancholic and melancholic. Nonmelancholic depression is more common, accounting for 90 percent of all cases. Symptoms come on gradually but typically emerge in the first four weeks after birth. This kind of postnatal depression is thought to be related to a reaction to stress rather than a biochemical imbalance.

Melancholic depression occurs in the remaining 10 percent of cases. It tends to be more serious, with a deeper and more pervasive depression that the mother is often unaware of. Symptoms, including reduced physical activity and joylessness, typically first appear in the first four weeks after birth.

How will your doctor come to a diagnosis of depression? The doctor will check in with you regarding your physical well-being, ask how you are coping, and likely administer a ten-question questionnaire called the EPDS (Edinburgh Postnatal Depression Scale) or an equivalent. If you are scoring above ten, the doctor may want to monitor or review you, and if you score above thirteen, you are likely to be referred to a specialist in postpartum depression.

Recent research by scientists in Australia has shown that the peak incidence of depression postnatally doesn't come within the first year after birth but happens *four years later*! This astonishing fact means that, for these sufferers, there is obviously a cumulative effect and that this depression is not just the result of the birth and hormonal changes. This is why if you have persistent symptoms of depression that come on after the birth of your baby, at the very least you need a thorough medical exam and testing of your hormones and micronutrient levels to see if depletion is a trigger.

THE BIGGEST KEY BETWEEN BEING DEPLETED AND BEING DEPRESSED

Symptoms of overlap that occur in both depletion and depression include sleep disturbances, fatigue, feelings of worthlessness and guilt, an inability to think clearly and concentrate, and/or significant weight change up or down.

One symptom that distinguishes depression from depletion is anhedo-

SLEEP DEPRIVATION AFFECTS NEW DADS, TOO

In my opinion, sleep deprivation can be one of the risk factors affecting new *dads* as well. Recent research published in Australia has shown that postpartum depression hits fathers and mothers at similar rates in the first twelve months after birth—occurring at a rate of one in ten dads and one in seven mothers. The major risk factor for a dad having depression is the mother's also having depression. I don't think this is just about the stress of caring for a baby but about a lack of parenthood preparedness, support, and a healthy dialogue about the new roles both parents need to process. I've heard from many of my patients that the complex changes in a new family are incredibly difficult to discuss, no matter how well both partners are otherwise able to communicate—so that what should be a catalyst for growth in the relationship (moving through the transition of romantic love to mature love) becomes instead a source of confusion, isolation, and eventually friction. New dads sometimes joke, "My wife has a new lover now... and that's the baby!" In these cases, bonding between mother and child is perceived as a source of alienation and frustration, especially as moms recovering from birth commonly have a nonexistent libido. If dads aren't prepared for these changes, the parents' relationship can suffer—sometimes irreparably.

Luckily Western society is changing, albeit slowly. Australian fathers are now the primary caregiver to their children in 10 percent of the families in this country, which is a huge increase over what was happening even five years ago. The better that moms and dads learn to share the child care, the more support they have, the more they are able to talk about their issues, the less likely depression will surface. And they'll get a lot more sleep, too!

nia, or the inability to derive pleasure from things that previously did bring pleasure. In depletion, despite your feeling dreadful, life at its core still feels good and it's possible to experience pleasure and enjoyment. In depression, there is no joy in the experience of motherhood and no enjoyment in activities or simple tasks that usually would have brought joy—going for a walk, cooking a good meal, seeing a sunset, laughing at a comedy. The deeper the depression, the less aware the depressed mother is of her depression as well.

Middle insomnia, in which a person has no difficulty falling asleep initially but significant trouble going back to sleep after awakening in the middle of the night, is another telltale symptom. It is common for a new mother to wake numerous times during the night, and the depleted mother will usually take a mere five minutes or so to fall back to sleep. The depressed mother, on the other hand, because of brain-chemical imbalance, can take up to one hour to fall back to sleep. She lies awake in the torment of overthinking and is consumed by negative thoughts, which typically occur during these dark hours.

In addition, symptoms that may indicate the condition of postnatal *anxiety* include initial insomnia, where it may take up to an hour for a mother to fall asleep, despite utter exhaustion. In these mothers there are often excessive concerns about their well-being, their baby's well-being, and their ability to cope.

Postpartum depression and anxiety can be extremely debilitating. Getting early support and follow-up from experienced medical professionals is essential. Typical treatments include counseling, support assessments, relationship support, advice about beneficial exercises, socialization, and, commonly, the use of antidepressants or antianxiety drugs. I am not opposed to pharmaceuticals. I will prescribe them at times myself and have seen them work wonderfully well. However, I am opposed to treatments in which these medications are the only support a mother is given. Obviously, I feel there is so much more, as discussed in this book, that can be done before a crisis of depression occurs.

It is important to know that postpartum depression is *not* a fixed destiny, and I see mothers recovering from this most of the time.

BABY BONDING AND HOW IT IMPACTS POSTNATAL DEPLETION

When I was a student training at the Auckland School of Medicine, I had an after-hours job for a year at a private maternity hospital. This was a small hospital that was exceptionally well run, and much care was given to providing a safe, supportive environment for mothers to birth in. This job was, however, far from glamorous—my primary tasks were to clean the patients' rooms and bathrooms and work in the kitchen. Another of my duties was bringing the daily meals to the mothers with their newborns. Not exactly the medical training I was expecting!

At this point, my only other experience with newborns and their mothers had been at the maternity ward of Middlemore Hospital in South Auckland, a stereotypical teaching hospital with antiseptic halls, ugly lighting, and endless rounds being made by medical students and junior doctors who hadn't yet mastered the art of a sympathetic bedside manner. So I was heartened every single day I worked at the private maternity hospital, because what I saw in these quiet, uncluttered rooms was new moms being given the space, calm, and time they needed to enhance their bonding with their tiny infants.

Often, I was bringing these moms their first meal or cup of tea after their babies had been born. The love that was emanating from the mothers and their newborns was palpable, and the glow and gratitude I saw in these mothers was deeply touching. It was like seeing a ray of mother–baby sunshine. In my personal life and in my medical training up to that point, I'd never seen or felt anything like it—I was used to seeing patients who were ill and in pain. These moms were the only "patients" I had seen who were happy to be in the hospital.

As my medical training progressed, and even as I spent countless days training in different maternity wards and in the neonatal units, I missed seeing those beaming, joyful faces of the moms gazing at their newborns with pure, sweet adoration in their rooms. I came to understand that mother–baby sunshine came from the undisturbed bonding that these new families were being allowed to do—and how vitally important it was to prevent postnatal depletion. I became intrigued with what was happening physiologically with this bond. A big part of this is the hormone oxytocin.

Oxytocin is the hormone that causes the powerful uterine contractions during labor. Oxytocin isn't just crucial during the birth process; it also plays an important role in mother–baby bonding during breastfeeding, which is why it's often called the attachment hormone. Whenever you breastfeed, the baby stimulates sensory nerve endings on your nipple, causing a release of both oxytocin and prolactin from the mother's brain. The hormone prolactin then signals the release of milk from the breast tissue and calls for the breast tissue to produce more milk.

Oxytocin has effects not only on the mother's brain but also on the *baby's* brain via the breast milk. In many mammals, oxytocin is so crucial to mother–baby bonding that it can mean the difference between life and death for the newborn. In sheep, for example, there is a huge spike of oxytocin soon after the birth of the lambs, and this is what allows the ewes to recognize their babies' unique scent and literally have it imprinted in their brains. If a newborn lamb is removed during this oxytocin spike, which lasts approximately five minutes, and returned to the mother even a mere hour later, the mother will not recognize or bond with its own offspring and will simply ignore the baby.

This is called the window for bonding. There is a sensitive period for several hours during the onset of labor in which oxytocin and prolactin receptors in the brain and in the breasts of the mother are primed for bonding with her newborn. If the natural cascade of hormones during child bearing does not occur, then what is created is described by experts as a "hormone gap." This hormone gap is widened if the mother has an elective C-section and, to a lesser degree, if she's given an epidural. Researchers are showing, however, that this hormone gap can be reduced and potentially corrected with early skin-to-skin contact and/or breastfeeding. Skin-to-skin time with mother and baby has even been shown to reduce rates of depression and increase survival rates of prematurely born babies.

Mothers often experience this as something akin to a "baby bubble"—they can actually feel that their "being" extends to include the baby—and this is often a source of profound wonderment. My partner, Caroline, fondly recalls this "sixth sense" that she felt with the arrival of our first child, Felix. She told me she was able to feel things that Felix was feeling, such as being hot or cold, without her feeling hot or cold herself. Other moms may recognize this feeling, as their breasts will start to leak milk the instant their baby starts to cry.

It is important that we respect this window of time for the bonding to occur between a mother and her newborn. It's equally important to understand the mother's heightened perceptions that lead to her being vigilant, hyperaware, highly emotional, and totally focused on her new baby. The reason for this is obvious, but it is a design that can be easily derailed by the modern approach to birthing and mothering. When this bonding doesn't take place, postnatal depletion can be even more debilitating.

WHAT HAPPENS IF YOU MISSED THE WINDOW FOR BONDING?

Some women have difficult and traumatic births, leaving them physically unable to see or touch their newborns for hours or even days. Sometimes babies who are born prematurely or with difficulties might be whisked off to the neonatal intensive care unit for intensive treatment in incubators.

I've had many moms in my clinic who were distraught at the circumstances of their babies' births and despondent that they didn't have the opportunity to have a normal birth and time together to bond afterward. I always tell them that it is *never* their fault and that there is a lot that mothers and families can do to heal these traumas and reconnect to their children. Children by nature are very forgiving, and when they come to experience love, support, and contact with their caregivers, they will flourish. Mothers must be given the validation they need to know that they were not "failures" if things didn't go as planned, or if choices were taken away from them during the birth due to unforeseen circumstances, or if they felt otherwise robbed of an idyllic baby-bonding phase that they see so often in the media.

Don't expect an apology from the hospital system, but if acknowledgment and sharing can happen through friends, families, mothers' groups, and/or counseling, moms can feel so much better. I see a lot of mothers gain great solace by working with a health-care provider who has experience in birth trauma. This can come in the form of a psychologist, counselor, midwife, or doula. By helping mothers explore these deep issues and by helping reframe a mother's experience, these health-care providers can support new moms in reconnecting with their role as mothers. If these issues remain unresolved, festering resentment or guilt can hinder a mother from developing in her role as a parent. Acknowledgment is the first step in finding resolution.

Our firstborn was quite an unsettled baby in the first year; he cried a lot and didn't sleep much. I remember the anxiety that Caroline experienced and how at 3:00 a.m. this could become a cascade. Even with all my medical knowledge and experience in the neonatal unit, as a father it was difficult not to worry that something was wrong with either the baby or how we were parenting.

We have emotions for a reason, and they should not be ignored or suppressed. They certainly should not be feared or hidden, particularly while the body is recovering from and reacting to the birth of a child. There's an enormous amount going on that can cause confusing or even unwelcome feelings, and there is nobody to blame for that. They will pass, with time and support—support in the home, support in the mind, and support in the heart. Emotions need to be acknowledged. Don't be hard on yourself. For emotional beings to have strength, we need restoration and support: restoration of the body, physically and emotionally. If you're struggling with emotions that make you uncomfortable, honor them and know that there is a path forward.

PART II

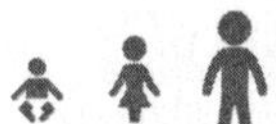

One Hundred Days of Repletion: Rebuilding Physical Wellness

I am constantly in awe of this thing that is the human body. With all its complexities, inherent intelligence, and self-modifying strategies, the workings of the human body are nearly beyond comprehension. Everything that happens inside—from how our cells process nutrients to how our organs function, our tissues get repaired, and our hormones send off signals telling everything what to do—is like an intricate and beautifully woven spider's web. You can't pull down one part of the web without affecting in some tiny or even some monumental way other parts of it. A single nutrient or hormone deficiency has widespread effects on how your beautiful web can function.

The flip side to this, of course, is that when you start to replenish specific nutrients that have been depleted, the entire net becomes even stronger and more beautiful. When you start to improve one part of the body, you improve every other part as well.

This idea is the heart of my program to end your depletion. The concept is to tackle biological depletion first, then psychological depletion. It's the same idea behind airlines' requiring that you position your own oxygen mask first before helping someone else put on theirs; to be useful to others, you must take care of yourself first.

When I coach patients about their health and wellness, I introduce them to the "Four Pillars of Health": sleep, purpose, activity, and nutrition (SPAN). These four pillars, or components, are integral to our "health span"—the part of our life when we are active, independent, and mercifully free of a debilitating disease. Ideally, our health span should match our life span as closely as possible. However, over recent decades, while there has been a slow increase in our life span, there has not been a corresponding increase in our *health* span.

As a medical student, I had a jaded view of aging. I believed that when we got older we were pretty much certain to fall victim to any number of chronic diseases and ailments, which would need a shelf full of prescribed medications to treat. Fortunately, I had an experience during my first year as a junior doctor that radically changed my perspective. It happened when I was doing an ophthalmology run. I needed to spend two afternoons a week manning the preadmission clinic for eye surgery. These clinics were typically busy, with only a certain amount of time allocated per patient. On one particular afternoon I saw that there were three ninety-year-olds on the patient list for the clinic, and I shook my head in disbelief. What a nightmare my afternoon was going to be! I was sure that I'd have to spend all afternoon calling nursing homes, trying to track down accurate lists of medications for these patients—and this task alone would eat up all their allotted time. How would I do this *and* take their medical history *and* examine them? Having one ninety-year-old was sure to slow things down, but having *three* was going to be impossible.

Well, was I in for a much-needed shock. Each of these elderly patients was leading a full, active life. Not one of them was on any prescribed medications. In fact, one of them had never before been to a hospital as a patient, apart from when he was born. One of them had made an appointment only to get his cataracts "dealt with" so he could go back to bush-walking (the Australian equivalent of hiking in the wilderness) with his friends. He was in and out of my office in just a few minutes, and I remember feeling both astonished and very ashamed of myself for having been so judgmental.

I went home on time that afternoon and spent that evening—and many, many more!—reevaluating my assumptions and slowly figuring out how to integrate what I had learned from those wise, witty, and very healthy ninety-year-olds into my expanding view of wellness. Eventually, I came up with the Four Pillars of Health; these are the components of wellness you'll try to balance as you recover from your postnatal depletion.

SPAN: THE FOUR PILLARS OF HEALTH

---

1. *S* Is for Sleep

You learned about sleep in chapter 2, and you know how important it is for all aspects of your well-being. (Chapter 8 will give you all the strategies you need so you can sleep well again.)

2. *P* Is for Purpose

This pillar is about ensuring that you feel connected to your place and role in the world and that you're engaged in your day-to-day life. Being able to identify your own personal mission statement and feel like you're making steps toward it is an essential part of experiencing peace and happiness. After all, if you can't state what makes you happy, how can you *be* happy?

It's equally important to feel like you are a contributing member of a community that allows you to explore and express the true nature of your self. There is no right or wrong way to do this; self-inquiry can take the form of religion, life coaching, yoga, martial arts, meditation, self-help groups, online forums, community involvement, or even simply regular conversation with a trusted friend or partner.

3. *A* Is for Activity

Human beings are meant to move. That's what we've been programmed to do over the course of our evolution, and this is what we need to do right now. Movement is an essential part of being healthy, as it helps get blood and oxygen to your cells as well as stimulates the flow of your lymph fluid from your cells. Movement includes posture, core strength, alignment, and a good walking style.

4. *N* Is for Nutrition

Doubtless you've heard the famous maxims "You are what you eat" and "Let food be thy medicine." Food is important because it nourishes your body and provides the ingredients and triggers for many of your most important physical functions. What you eat determines the amount of energy you have and your ability to focus and sleep.

But the issue of food is complex, and it covers not just what you eat but also how and when you eat (and this includes the social aspects of sitting down to a meal). Understanding what, how, and when you eat is a critical step in being able to care for yourself—and your family.

In the following chapters, I show you the easy steps you can take to move from depletion to repletion. You'll learn in chapter 4 how to increase your levels of micronutrients (vitamins and minerals). Chapter 5 addresses the replacement of macronutrients (specific proteins and amino acids, specific fats, and, to a lesser degree, carbohydrates). Once there's a reasonable balance between your improved micronutrient and macronutrient levels, your organs will start to function better. The most important organs in the postnatal period include the liver, brain, and intestines. Once organ function is improved, you'll get to work on replenishing your hormones.

The good news is that what you'll need to do to improve your hormonal health is minimalized once you improve your micro- and macronutrient status and organ function. You'll see that there is a lot of overlap in the repletion categories. One hundred percent improvement in one category isn't necessary before you move on to the next.

CHAPTER 4

Rebuilding Micronutrients

Repletion is all about improving the internal environment of your body so you can restore what went missing when you became depleted. When you look at the process of pregnancy, childbirth, and breastfeeding, your body's demand for micronutrients—vitamins and minerals—is huge. Add in the stress of sleep deprivation, which through hormonal reasons can add to your depleted load, and you will have a big "debt" of micronutrients to pay back. The placenta seems to show preferential treatment to the developing fetus when it comes to micronutrients and macronutrients. Whatever the baby needs, the mother supplies... often leaving her lacking enough for herself.

The very first step in your repletion plan is to rebuild your micronutrients. I've found that if you don't do this first, it will be much harder for you to improve your hormone levels.

Because replenishing a single nutrient has only limited effects, my clinic creates individualized plans in which a particular sequence of multiple supplements will build on one another. I don't want the mothers I treat to have to take supplements for life—the goal is to create a strong new foundation to build from and let the body take it from there, which *does* happen. Once your depletion is on its way to being cured, you'll be able to get the micronutrients you need from the nutrient-dense foods you'll read about in chapter 9.

Why Supplements?

I recommend and prescribe supplements. Of course, it's also important to eat foods that are rich in nutrition and the specific vitamins and minerals you are looking to increase. But there is a loss of mineral and vitamin density in food due to poor soil mineral content and long-term storage of foods. Foods are thus good at maintaining levels but can be poor at replacing levels of minerals and vitamins.

HOW CELLS WORK AND HOW MICRONUTRIENTS HELP THEM WORK PROPERLY

Micronutrients are the vitamins and minerals that help regulate our metabolism. They are needed for healthy growth and development and are found in the foods we eat and, with vitamin D, in the rays from the sun. They are called micronutrients because you need only a very small amount of them.

Some vitamins are water soluble, meaning that you excrete the excess in your urine and need to replace them regularly. Others are fat soluble, meaning that they are used in cell membranes and can be stored in your fat when you don't need them.

Think of your body as a city that's made up of all different sizes of LEGO pieces. Some of the pieces are small; others are large and sturdy. LEGO pieces are designed so they easily interconnect and can be used to build bigger things, like houses. Micronutrients are like the very smallest LEGO pieces. They can't be broken down into even tinier pieces—only added on to larger pieces. But without them, you can't keep on building.

Your micronutrients get depleted in the process of making, birthing, and feeding your baby. If they are not replaced, your depletion will worsen. And if you have a preexisting condition such as an autoimmune disease or intestinal absorption issues, replacing these micronutrients will be even harder. To rebuild, repair, and replace, we need these micronutrients not just in adequate amounts but also in a good balance in relation to one another.

Many women take prenatal multivitamins and mineral formulas and think that's enough. It isn't. Consider, for example, that an average steak contains about 6 mg iron, which is only one-third of the minimum recommended dietary allowance (RDA) for a healthy woman. Because iron is hard to absorb, many women are extremely deficient, and an average supplement won't fix the problem. These prenatal supplements are designed with a conservative average in mind and are based on the minimum dose needed for preventing diseases in the fetus (e.g., spina bifida, cretinism, and rickets). In other words, they're all about ensuring that *the baby* is healthy, but they do not provide enough micronutrients for the mother's optimal functioning. That's why these supplements often fall short of what you actually need to deal with your depletion. You will see that what I recommend can be many times above the RDA. (To learn which foods are rich in particular micronutrients, which will add to the levels in the supplements you're taking, see chapter 9.)

Taking handfuls of pills can also be counterproductive unless you know what levels to take and in which combinations. If, for example, you take a B-complex supplement when you are actually low in zinc, manganese, molybdenum, and selenium, you won't get the benefits you are hoping for, and your body then has to get rid of what it doesn't need. What follows is my targeted strategy for identifying and restoring specific depleted nutrients.

ESSENTIAL MICRONUTRIENTS

When you have postnatal depletion, these are the important micronutrients you need to restore, in descending order of importance. Using the checklists in this chapter will help you pinpoint any deficiencies/excess you are currently experiencing.

1. Iron
2. Zinc
3. Vitamin B_{12}
4. Vitamin D

5. Copper
6. Magnesium
7. Trace elements, including iodine, selenium, molybdenum, and manganese
8. Other B vitamins
9. Vitamin C
10. Fat-soluble vitamins, especially vitamins A, E, and K_2

1. *Iron*

This all-important mineral is crucial for the function of more than one hundred proteins and enzymes in your body. It helps with the energy-production process in your cells, protects your body against oxidation, and assists your liver in breaking down toxins. And it has a very important role as the center of the heme complex, which makes hemoglobin, the molecule that carries oxygen within your red blood cells.

Without enough iron, you'll be tired and lacking your usual energy, and your cells won't be getting enough oxygen. You may not even have enough red blood cells; this common condition in people who are iron deficient is called anemia. You might also notice that the sclera (the white part of your eyes) has a slight blush tinge to it and that the palmar creases (the deeper grooves on the surface of your palms) are a very light color.

A complicating issue with iron has to do with its absorption. I actually call this a design fault that we humans have, as we can only absorb food-based iron in the first few inches of the small intestine as it exits from the stomach. Worse, no matter what we eat, on average we can absorb only about 18 percent of the iron from animal sources and only about 10 percent of the iron from plant sources. And if you don't chew your food extremely well or if your stomach acids are low (meaning you don't digest your food efficiently), you will have even more trouble getting the iron absorption you need. The minimum RDA (recommended dietary allowance) for a healthy woman with no postnatal depletion is 18 mg. We can at best absorb between 10 and 30 mg iron per day, so this means that if someone is severely deficient in iron it can take months of oral supplements and iron-rich foods to get iron levels even close to optimal.

To give you examples of iron amounts in food, 2½ ounces beef has 2.4 mg iron; ½ cup cooked spinach has 3.4 mg; and 1 cup raw spinach has 0.9 mg. Those numbers are nowhere close to tackling your iron depletion.

How to Test for Iron Deficiency

A blood test will easily diagnose iron deficiency as long as you have a clinician who looks for iron levels in the optimal range. Iron levels are a good example of how people can suffer when a laboratory reference range and a biological optimal range have nothing to do with each other. By definition, most laboratory reference ranges have to include 95 percent of the results within that range. So to have iron deficiency according to lab ranges, you need to be in the bottom 2.5 percent of the population—yet studies show that in Australia up to 25 percent of the population is iron deficient. This means that about one in five people blood-tested for iron is told that her results are normal when they are actually deficient.

You want your ferritin (the iron-storage molecule) level to be at approximately 50 mcg/L. If it is lower than 25 mcg/L, you should assume that you are iron deficient and start treating it immediately.

Quick Test for Iron Deficiency

To score: Never = 0, Sometimes = 1, Always = 2

Iron	Never	Sometimes	Always
Do you struggle to think clearly or frequently feel confused?			
Do you have difficulty concentrating?			
Do your muscles get tired easily?			
Do you get breathless easily?			
Have you had low iron or been anemic in the past?			

Iron	Never	Sometimes	Always
Do you get restless legs?			
Do you feel the cold easily?			
Do you have brittle hair?			
Are you experiencing hair loss?			
Do you have brittle nails?			
Are your nails flat or spoon shaped?			
Do you suffer from heavy periods?			
Do you have a thyroid condition?			
Do you suffer from cracks or sores in the corners of your mouth?			
Do you have a painful red and swollen tongue?			
Do you suffer from mood swings and irritability?			
Do you struggle with fatigue?			
Do you suffer with frequent or recurrent infections (of any type)?			

Iron score: 14 or more = Iron insufficiency or deficiency possible; more than 22 = Iron insufficiency or deficiency very likely.

How to Treat Iron Deficiency

The minimum RDA for iron is 18 mg for a healthy adult woman, 27 mg for a pregnant woman, and 9 mg for a nonmenstruating, breastfeeding mother. (No, these numbers are not wrong. Although it does seem strange that a breastfeeding mother should need only half the amount of iron of someone who isn't nourishing a baby, a woman who isn't menstruating isn't losing as much iron as someone who is.) In my clinic, we often fast-track iron repletion with intravenous infusions of iron. We use only iron sucrose due to its high safety profile and its tolerability. These infusions usually start to work within a few days or, if someone is very deficient, up to a few weeks. I am always thrilled when my patients get their energy back and are far less fatigued. After we have restored iron levels, then mothers will often switch to an oral supplement to help maintain iron levels while we focus on other areas of recovery.

Obviously, you can't do this on your own. Have your blood tested for iron and if your ferritin level is under 25 mcg/L, supplements such as iron glycinate can help you. The new generation of iron supplements are easily absorbed throughout the digestive tract and do not have the typical side effects of constipation, dark stools, and nausea.

2. *Zinc*

Zinc is a big player in your body's overall functioning. It's a cofactor in more than three hundred enzymes and is needed so that these enzymes function properly. (An enzyme is a protein that has a specific function in your body.) The list of tasks that the zinc-requiring enzymes perform is long, but for postnatally depleted mothers its most important chores involve promoting digestive health, keeping the immune system strong so it can fight off infections, synthesizing DNA, making the brain's neurotransmitters (chemical messengers), and regulating hormones.

As with iron, there is an inherent absorption problem with zinc. Zinc is needed to make stomach acids, but you need to have enough stomach acids before you can absorb zinc properly. This is a perfect example of the slippery slope you find yourself sliding down in which depletion begets depletion!

How to Test for Zinc Deficiency

A plasma zinc level is a reasonable test for your doctor to conduct to determine how much zinc your body has available (like cash in your wallet), but it doesn't look at body stores that can't be used due to other nutrient imbalances (like cash in a frozen bank account). This is why blood tests every six to twelve weeks may be required to assess improvements in your zinc levels and its metabolism. I prefer a plasma zinc level of at least 15 umol/L or above. Below 15 umol/L indicates insufficiency. Below 10 umol/L indicates a very significant deficiency.

Quick Test for Zinc Deficiency

To score: Never = 0, Sometimes = 1, Always = 2

Zinc	Never	Sometimes	Always
Do you get white spots on your nails?			
Have you noticed reduced taste or smell?			
Do you suffer from anxiety or nervousness?			
Do you have difficulty concentrating?			
Do you find wounds take a long time to heal?			
Has your night vision deteriorated?			
Are your eyes very sensitive to light?			
Do you suffer from sore, inflamed eyes?			
Do you get a tremor in your hand or fingers when you try to press a button or touch a finger to the tip of your nose?			
Do you experience "skin rashes"?			
Do you suffer from diarrhea?			
Do you suffer from cracks or sores in the corners of your mouth?			
Do you experience poor appetite, especially for breakfast?			
Do you experience feelings of depression that can last for more than a few hours?			
Do you suffer with frequent or recurrent infections (of any type)?			
Are you experiencing hair loss?			
Would others say that you have a short fuse to getting angry or irritable?			
Did you have many stretch marks from pregnancy?	None	Several	Many

Zinc score: 12 or more = Zinc insufficiency or deficiency possible; 18 or more = Zinc insufficiency or deficiency very likely.

How to Treat Zinc Deficiency

The minimum RDA for zinc is 8 mg for a healthy adult woman, 11 mg for a pregnant woman, and 12 mg for a breastfeeding mother. Studies have shown that 82 percent of pregnant women worldwide don't get enough zinc. For patients with low levels of zinc, I recommend a baseline dose of 25 mg zinc picolinate or zinc citrate as a replacement dose as opposed to the suggested maintenance doses mentioned earlier. I recheck zinc every three months. The only long-term downside of zinc supplements is the potential for reducing copper stores—which as you will see in the "Copper" section is not a bad outcome, as a majority of my postnatally depleted mothers have too much free copper in their systems.

3. *Vitamin B_{12}*

Vitamin B_{12} is vitally important for building, repairing, and detoxifying during energy production as well as aiding in healthy immune function. It also helps protect our DNA from damage. Vitamin B_{12} is the largest and most complex of all the vitamins (and I believe it should stand alone rather than being unceremoniously lumped together with all the other B vitamins).

Vitamin B_{12} not only comes from food sources but can also be made by bacteria in your gut, so anything that affects your bacteria can easily affect its production, too. If you also have low levels of stomach acid, this can further compromise B_{12} absorption. In addition, if you have high levels of copper along with low levels of vitamin B_{12}, this is a big contributor to your wooly-thinking, short-term-memory brain fog.

How to Test for Vitamin B_{12} Deficiency

A blood level for vitamin B_{12} and/or active B_{12} is a good screening test. A more accurate test is looking at your MMA (methylmalonic acid) level in either your blood or urine. If a patient's brain fog isn't improving despite initial treatment, I will sometimes do a urinary organic acids

(UOA) test, but this interpretation is not straightforward and only a highly trained health practitioner can do a proper assessment.

Quick Test for Vitamin B_{12} Deficiency

To score: Never = 0, Sometimes = 1, Always = 2

Vitamin B_{12}	Never	Sometimes	Always
Do you have a painful red and swollen tongue?			
Do you have smooth red patches on your tongue (called geographic tongue)?			
Do you suffer from diarrhea or stomach pains?			
Do you have a malabsorption disease (e.g., celiac disease)?			
Have you noticed changes in your personality?			
Have you noticed increased forgetfulness?			
Do you struggle to think clearly or frequently feel confused?			
Have you noticed increased clumsiness or poor coordination?			
Do you have patches of darker skin on your face, neck, or arms (hyperpigmentation)?			
Do you experience heart palpitations in which your heart is beating too hard or too fast, skipping a beat, or fluttering?			
Do you get dizzy when you stand up?			
Do you experience numbness, tingling, or weakness in your arms or legs?			
Do you take a proton-pump inhibitor medication like Nexium?			
Do you take Metformin (a diabetes drug)?			
Do you have a poor appetite?			
Do you struggle with fatigue?			

Vitamin B_{12}	Never	Sometimes	Always
Do you suffer with frequent or recurrent infections (of any type)?			
Do you experience feelings of depression that can last for more than a few hours?			
Do you find yourself easily irritated?			

B_{12} score: 14 or more = Vitamin B_{12} insufficiency or deficiency possible; 25 or more = Vitamin B_{12} insufficiency or deficiency very likely.

How to Treat Vitamin B_{12} Deficiency

The minimum RDA for B_{12} is 2.4 pg for a healthy adult woman, 2.6 pg for a pregnant woman, and 2.8 pg for a breastfeeding mother. If vitamin B_{12} is low, I usually recommend either a single intramuscular injection of methyl B_{12} (10 mg) or a sublingual spray of liposomal methyl B_{12} (1,000 mcg) daily for one month. Remember, once your stores of vitamin B_{12} are restored, your body can remain topped up for up to 2 years.

4. *Vitamin D*

Vitamin D is responsible for increasing the intestinal absorption of calcium, iron, magnesium, phosphate, and zinc. It also plays a significant role in how your body processes calcium. The best-known manifestations of vitamin D deficiency is rickets in children and osteoporosis in adults, caused by an inadequate mineralization of the bones. In other words, these bones get soft or brittle.

Good, strong bones are not the only part of your body that needs vitamin D—nearly all of your body's cells have vitamin D_3 receptors, which help increase how rapidly these cells get their work done. For this, vitamin D actually acts like a hormone, sending out signals to cells. The result is that it helps increase genetic expression, which is critical in controlling inflammation. In other words, the better the vitamin D, the better and more quickly information can get into the cells. This really is a big deal, especially when you're depleted.

How to Test for Vitamin D Deficiency

A blood test looking at the 25-OH form of vitamin D gives a good indication of how much vitamin D is stored in your body.

Quick Test for Vitamin D Deficiency

To score: Never = 0, Sometimes = 1, Always = 2

Vitamin D	Never	Sometimes	Always
Do you suffer from muscle pain?			
Do you suffer from bone pain?			
Do you suffer from osteoporosis?			
Do you suffer from muscle weakness in the thighs or upper arms?			
Do you suffer from chronic lower-back ache?			
Do you suffer from high blood sugar levels?			
Does your scalp sweat?			
Have you noticed your skin is more sensitive to touch (hyperesthesia)?			
Do you suffer with frequent or recurrent infections (of any type)?			

Vitamin D score: 5 or more = Vitamin D deficiency possible; 10 or more = Vitamin D deficiency likely.

How to Treat Vitamin D Deficiency

The minimum RDA for vitamin D is 400 IU for a healthy adult woman, 600 IU for a pregnant woman, and 600 IU for a breastfeeding mother. For vitamin D deficiency, I recommend a much higher replacement dose at 5,000 units (IU) of vitamin D for six weeks and then a retest. Women who are severely deficient (20 ng/ml or 50 nmol/L) should talk to a doctor about the possibility of an intramuscular injection of 600,000 IU of vitamin D, which usually lasts for a year.

You can make vitamin D from the sun's UVB rays, but I'll bet you didn't know the sun needs to be at least 45 degrees to the horizon to make sufficient vitamin D. (There are apps available that actually tell you the angle of the sun in your area so you can maximize exposure. The best known is Dminder.) To avoid skin damage from the sun, I usually recommend getting fifteen to twenty minutes of sun with the face protected (we don't make much vitamin D on our faces) and the belly and thighs exposed. The belly and thighs are our body's solar panels, where we make most of our vitamin D, so it is better to expose them to the sun than it is to bare your arms or calves. You can make 20,000 IU of vitamin D this way, and I recommend three sessions like this per week. After those fifteen to twenty minutes, cover up or apply a high SPF sunscreen.

Do *not* get into water or shower for at least ten minutes after your fifteen- to twenty-minute sun exposure, as you can literally wash off the vitamin D that has just formed on the surface of your skin! If you burn easily, then supplements are a better source of vitamin D than the sun.

5. *Copper*

Copper is a mysterious mineral that helps balance our oxidation rate due to its use by many important enzymes. It is also needed for making red blood cells and blood vessels. Obviously this is important for pregnancy and placentas, where blood and blood vessels need to be made at a fast rate. And because the female hormone estrogen has an effect on retaining copper, it is much easier for women to accumulate copper than it is for men. During pregnancy, serum copper levels should typically double from 110 mcg/dL to 220 mcg/dL, with copper and estrogen levels usually dropping within twenty-four hours after delivery of the baby. But studies have shown that women who have postnatal depression often do not have this drop in copper levels. Some researchers believe that this is a *cause* of postpartum depression, but until more research is done, I see it more as an amplifier of the symptoms of depression.

Copper deficiency, like iron deficiency, classically causes anemia and is related to malabsorption, but I see this very rarely. The more common issue postnatally is that of copper excess, which leads to some important consequences.

First, high copper levels have a deleterious effect on two of your brain chemicals in particular: noradrenaline and dopamine. Noradrenaline is the neurotransmitter that prepares your brain to receive and respond to stimuli from the environment; it makes you vigilant. However, too much of it, which high copper levels can cause, will turn vigilance to anxiety. High copper levels also reduce dopamine, which regulates pleasure and well-being and is often implicated in cases of obsessive, addictive, and compulsive behaviors. (We get a release of dopamine every time we connect to social media—it's what keeps us hooked on Facebook!) When dopamine levels drop, we become less engaged and excited about our interests, leading to depression.

Second, too much copper acts as a potent pro-oxidant in the body, causing inflammation. It oxidizes vitamin C, reduces progesterone levels in the second half of your menstrual cycle, and indirectly reduces iron absorption, contributing to fatigue. Zinc and magnesium don't work as well when copper levels are too high. Copper also blocks carnitine production, which is important for energy production and burning fat; carnitine deficiency is associated with poor sleep and increased sugar cravings.

My comment to patients is that excess copper will make whatever problems you have worse: if you are prone to headaches, your headaches will be worse; if you have eczema, it will make your eczema worse. Lowering levels to normal will help you feel a lot better in many different ways, especially when dopamine levels are corrected, as you'll find it easier to self-regulate your emotions. You'll feel less overwhelmed, better in your own skin, and more confident and capable of tackling motherhood's many challenges.

How to Test for Copper Excess/Deficiency

The diagnosis of copper toxicity is not straightforward and requires analysis of the plasma zinc level, the serum copper level, and the copper-carrying protein, ceruloplasmin. A free copper level of 25 percent or higher indicates copper excess; the ideal level is 20 percent or below.

You should also have your zinc levels tested, as copper and zinc act like brother and sister. They don't necessarily get along, but they do tolerate each other when their levels are equal. However, low zinc levels can make the effects of high copper even worse. A copper-to-zinc ratio greater than one indicates excess copper. Many women with excess copper tend to get itchy skin or a greenish tint to their skin if they are wearing any inexpensive jewelry that's made from nickel; they can tolerate only gold and silver. If this happens to you, get your copper tested!

Quick Test for Copper Excess

To score: Never = 0, Sometimes = 1, Always = 2

Copper Overload/Excess	Never	Sometimes	Always
Do you experience skin sensitivity to nickel (e.g., itch, rash, or discoloration from "cheap" jewelry)?			
Do you experience tinnitus (a ringing sensation in your ears)?			
Do you find yourself feeling anxious?			
Have you ever had an adverse reaction (e.g., nausea, headache) from taking a mineral supplement?			
Are you prone to emotional meltdowns?			
Do you have problems going to sleep or staying asleep?			

Copper excess score: 4 or more = Copper excess possible; 7 or more = Copper excess very likely.

How to Treat Copper Excess/Deficiency

Treatment for copper excess typically consists of six weeks of "zinc loading" and then, while continuing the zinc, adding the trace element molybdenum. There can be a mild worsening of symptoms at around ten days after starting treatment, with improvement usually occurring between three and four weeks later and a full effect occurring three to four months later. This lessens the copper levels.

Because the problem with copper is its excess, I've rarely had to treat a patient for a copper deficiency. The minimum RDA for copper is 900 mcg for a healthy adult woman, and I would expect most women to exceed that level.

6. *Magnesium*

Magnesium is the "mama" mineral, or "mom-nesium." I call it this because, as in a big family, the mama makes sure everything gets done and at the right pace. Without magnesium, nothing works quite right; magnesium doesn't get the credit it deserves in the world of nutritional medicine. The proper functioning of calcium, iron, zinc, and copper all depend on magnesium doing its job.

Magnesium is needed to support the energy cycles, to help your muscles move fluidly and your nerves function, to enhance sleep by increasing melatonin production, to improve the release of your brain chemicals, to stabilize blood sugar, to support bone health, and to support the production of DHEA (dehydroepiandrosterone), an adrenal steroid hormone that helps with energy stability.

If your magnesium levels are depleted, your symptoms will include fatigue, muscle tension, agitation, poor and light sleep with early-morning waking, poor concentration and memory, and fuzzy and agitated brain function.

Your body is not good at holding on to magnesium, and stress will cause you to excrete more of it in your urine.

How to Test for Magnesium Deficiency

This common nutrient is one of the hardest to accurately test for. Blood tests will show if it's low, but you can still have a significant deficiency with normal blood levels. The best test, and one that's underused and requires appropriate interpretation, is a twenty-four-hour urinary minerals assessment. Frustratingly, high levels of free copper will block your body's ability to use magnesium. I've found that a low twenty-four-hour urinary magnesium level combined with a low-normal corrected calcium level on a blood test indicates a profound magnesium deficiency.

Quick Test for Magnesium Deficiency

To score: Never = 0, Sometimes = 1, Always = 2

Magnesium	Never	Sometimes	Always
Do you suffer from muscle cramps or spasms?			
Do you have trouble sleeping?			
Do you suffer from anxiety or panic attacks?			
Do you suffer from irritability?			
Have you noticed increased forgetfulness?			
Do you have difficulty concentrating?			
Do you struggle to think clearly or frequently feel confused?			
Do you experience muscle shaking or trembling (tremor)?			
Do you experience heart palpitations in which your heart is beating too hard or too fast, skipping a beat, or fluttering?			
Do you experience feelings of depression that can last for more than a few hours?			
Do you experience rapid breathing?			
Do you suffer from frequent headaches?			
Do you suffer from nausea or vomiting?			
Have you noticed changes in your personality?			
Do you have pain at the base of your neck?			
Do you struggle with fatigue?			
Do you experience poor appetite?			

Magnesium score: 10 or more = Magnesium insufficiency or deficiency possible; 20 or more = Magnesium insufficiency or deficiency very likely.

How to Treat Magnesium Deficiency

The minimum RDA for magnesium is 310 mg for a healthy adult woman, 320 mg for a pregnant woman, and 360 mg for a breastfeeding mother. Magnesium citrate, malate, and glycinate are great forms to help with energy during the day and relaxation during the night. I use doses of 400 to 500 mg elemental magnesium daily to help rebalance levels, and retest every three months. Using magnesium sulfate as bath salts or as a foot soak can be a fantastic way to relax, especially before bed (ten to twenty minutes is plenty). The skin, especially via the feet, can absorb very generous amounts of this wonderful magnesium.

7. *Trace Elements, Including Iodine, Selenium, Molybdenum, and Manganese*

Trace elements are like the specialty tradesmen—the plumbers, electricians, and carpenters—on a work site. They do specific and important jobs. If they are absent, then all the other workers just sit around waiting for instructions. The four most important trace elements that I see commonly depleted in the postnatal period are iodine, selenium, molybdenum, and manganese.

Iodine is needed for healthy hormone production, especially the thyroid hormones. It is important in proper immune function and vitally important for breast and ovarian health. Fibrocystic breast disorder, for example, often responds very well to iodine supplements.

Selenium is important in helping bring balance in cholesterol issues, thyroid disorders, and autoimmune conditions. It buffers against the effect of the ever-present exposure to heavy metals that we face.

Molybdenum has a unique role in improving iron storage and keeping copper levels in check. It also helps your body rid itself of toxins in the liver and in the gut. Fluoride inhibits absorption of molybdenum—low levels of fluoride are seen in patients with tooth decay. Low zinc and molybdenum levels can lead to an increase in copper absorption from your gut—resulting in the nutrient imbalance problems discussed in the "Copper" section.

Manganese is important for brain function and helps alleviate mood swings. The balance among copper, zinc, molybdenum, and manganese significantly affects how histamines are metabolized, which, in turn, affects allergies, skin rashes, and eczema. Low levels can lead to aching joints, worsening skin problems, and anxiety.

How to Test for Trace Elements Deficiency

A screening test for iodine is a spot urine test in the morning. A more definitive test is the twenty-four-hour iodine challenge test, which must be set up by a health practitioner. If you avoid seaweed and other iodine-containing foods for twenty-four hours before the spot test, it's usually sufficient. I prefer a level over 100 mcg/ml. For other trace elements, the best test is a twenty-four-hour urine collection, which will specifically measure all of them.

How to Treat Trace Elements Deficiency

The minimum RDA for iodine is 150 mcg for a healthy adult woman, 220 mcg for a pregnant woman, and 290 mcg for a breastfeeding mother. The minimum RDA for selenium is 55 mcg for a healthy adult woman, 60 mcg for a pregnant woman, and 70 mcg for a breastfeeding mother. The minimum RDA for molybdenum is 45 mcg for a healthy adult woman, 50 mcg for a pregnant woman, and 50 mcg for a breastfeeding mother. The minimum RDA for manganese is 5 mg for a healthy adult woman, 5 mg for a pregnant woman, and 5 mg for a breastfeeding mother.

I typically treat patients who have depleted trace elements with 100 to 200 mcg iodine daily; 100 to 200 mcg selenium daily; 200 to 300 mcg molybdenum daily; and 5 to 10 mg manganese daily. This may come as an over-the-counter multimineral supplement (usually called a trace minerals complex), which often has useful added levels of zinc and chromium. Alternatively, I might request an individualized prescription through a compounding pharmacy. Supplements are taken for 3 months and then levels are retested.

8. *Other B Vitamins*

The other B vitamins are like the worker bees in a hive—they all have their specific tiny jobs and are noticed only in their absence. We evolved in a world where B vitamins, apart from vitamin B_{12}, were always in abundance, and the body has no way of storing them.

B vitamins are involved in energy production and maintaining a healthy mood. To be useful, these vitamins need to be activated *inside* the cells, and the only way they can get in there is if you have adequate levels of zinc and all the other trace elements. Taking a B-complex supplement, as I mentioned earlier in this chapter, when you are low in zinc, manganese, molybdenum, and selenium will be ineffective and a waste of your money.

How to Test for Other B Vitamin Deficiencies

The B vitamins are best measured in the urinary organic acids (UOA) test. Vitamin B_9 (folate) can also be blood-tested.

How to Treat Other B Vitamin Deficiencies

The minimum RDA for B-group vitamins varies, and most people take a supplement that includes all of them, if needed. Usually, I recommend a general activated B-complex supplement. Look for one that has vitamin B_9 (folate) as folinic acid or 5-MTHF.

9. *Vitamin C*

This important vitamin has many roles. It's especially important for collagen synthesis, which keeps your skin, gums, and ligaments supple; the health of your adrenal hormones; and energy production, especially in your mitochondria. It is also an all-around vital antioxidant.

The highest concentration of vitamin C in the body is found in your adrenal gland, which produces the adrenal hormones cortisol and DHEA. These, as you likely know, are the hormones released when we are under stress, so it makes sense that when we are stressed, we need more vitamin C.

The second-highest concentration of vitamin C is found in the brain, where it is indispensable in the making of the important neurotransmitters dopamine, noradrenaline, serotonin, and melatonin.

How to Test for Vitamin C Deficiency

Vitamin C can be assessed only as part of the UOA test, looking specifically at the ascorbic acid level. If it's below 10 mmol/molCr, this indicates a significant deficiency.

How to Treat Vitamin C Deficiency

The minimum RDA for vitamin C is 75 mg for a healthy adult woman, 85 mg for a pregnant woman, and 120 mg for a breastfeeding mother. In my clinic, I typically recommend doses of 1,000 to 2,000 mg vitamin C daily for six to twelve weeks, depending on symptoms. Ideally, my patients transition from vitamin C oral supplements to foods that are high in vitamin C at around that time. An orange, for example, contains 70 mg vitamin C—nearly the complete RDA. If you take too much vitamin C, the only side effects you may get are gurgling intestines and loose stool.

10. *Fat-Soluble Vitamins: Vitamins A, E, and K_2*

Vitamin A is important for all your mucous membranes and their immune function as well as maintaining good vision.

Vitamin E is an antioxidant that keeps your cell membranes healthy.

Vitamin K_2 helps keep calcium in the right places by moving it around the body, into the bones and teeth and out of soft tissues such as arteries.

Remember—fat-soluble vitamins can't be excreted by your body, so they accumulate over time. Never take megadoses unless prescribed by your doctor.

How to Test for Fat-Soluble Vitamin Deficiencies

Vitamins A and E can easily be measured in a blood test. Vitamin K_2 can be measured in a special undercarboxylated osteocalcin (ucOc) test, but it is not easily available.

A common way to assess whether the fat-soluble vitamins may be low is to look at the teeth. If the two top front teeth, in particular, show an increased translucency, making them appear glassy at the very bottom, this is a good indication that supplementation is needed.

How to Treat Fat-Soluble Vitamin Deficiencies

The minimum RDA for vitamin A is 2,300 IU for a healthy adult woman, 2,700 IU for a pregnant woman, and 3,600 IU for a breastfeeding mother. When a patient is depleted, I recommend between 5,000 and 10,000 IU daily for up to six weeks at a time.

The minimum RDA for vitamin E is 10 IU for a healthy adult woman, 10 IU for a pregnant woman, and 15 IU for a breastfeeding mother. The dosage range is huge and needs to be individualized. For very depleted patients, I often prescribe up to 400 IU of vitamin E as mixed tocopherols for typically six weeks at a time.

The minimum RDA for vitamin K_2 is 60 mcg for a healthy adult woman, 60 mcg for a pregnant woman, and 60 mcg for a breastfeeding mother. It's usually easy to reach these amounts in the food you eat if you include free-range eggs, aged cheeses, and fermented foods. *Nattō*, or Japanese fermented soybeans, are particularly high in vitamin K_2.

WENDY'S REGIMEN

Wendy was thirty-two years old when she first starting seeing me. She'd been in good health up until the birth of her son, who had just turned two. She'd been a vegan for most of her adult life and came to see me mainly to improve her energy and her clarity of mind and to find balance. She told me that she'd wake zombie-like in the morning and never seemed to get any energy going as the morning went on. She would have an energy crash in the afternoon and slowly became more awake in the evening. Her memory recall and concentration were terrible, and she was worrying and overthinking "everything," as she put it. She also had neck pain and headaches, which she'd started getting a few weeks before she came to see me.

What the Testing Showed

My testing showed that Wendy had low levels of iron and homocysteine (an amino acid), and her zinc-to-copper ratio was out of whack.

Wendy's Protocol

Wendy had two infusions of iron; a specific solution of iron was injected intravenously over thirty minutes and then repeated a week later. She also took a multimineral, DHA supplement, and NAC (the amino acid n-acetylcysteine) every day. The iron infusions quickly improved Wendy's energy and concentration, and after six weeks she was vastly better. She was also referred to a physical therapist and acupuncturist, as well as a psychologist who specialized in postnatal issues. By three months she told me she was feeling the best she'd felt "in a long time."

I didn't see Wendy again for nearly two years. She came back to see me when she was thirty-two weeks pregnant with her next child. She joked that she'd felt so much better after our initial visits she decided to have another baby, because she knew she wouldn't have to worry about her energy or brain fog anymore! Still, although she was in much better shape than the very first time I'd seen her, she was starting to get tired, wasn't sleeping well, and was waking up very irritable, which was something she'd never felt before. She wanted to get going on treatments as she didn't want to wait until she was feeling as bad as when she'd first come to see me.

Her iron, vitamin D, and cortisol levels were low, so I treated her with two iron infusions and one injection of intramuscular vitamin B_{12} and restarted the same oral multimineral supplement and DHA along with ashwagandha, an Ayurvedic herb. For sleep, I told her to take no more than one nap for up to twenty minutes each day, even if she wanted to sleep more, and to reduce her exposure to blue light at night. I also advised her to take supplements of liposomal curcumin and magnesium before bed.

Wendy came to see me four weeks later and she told me she was feeling wonderful. She was sleeping well, she had no more irritability when she woke up, and her energy had improved. She was looking forward to the birth of her second child. All went well, and whenever I see her pushing her baby in the stroller, she tells me she's loving life and her role as a busy mom. For the longer term, the only supplement Wendy is taking is ashwagandha.

You can see how little Wendy actually needed in terms of micronutrient supplementation to make an enormous difference in her energy and well-being. I hope your results will be just as spectacular.

JENNIFER'S REGIMEN

Jennifer was thirty-two, and her children were four and two and a half when she came to see me. She told me she was lethargic and had sleep problems, frequent headaches, a sore throat, cold sores, and frequent skin infections. She was also bothered by "overthinking everything." She'd had two traumatic births with emergency C-sections and felt she'd missed out and been disempowered by her experiences in the hospital—and she didn't want a repeat for the third child she and her husband were planning. With her first birth, Jennifer told me that she'd been pressured into having a C-section, and no one took the time to explain why, what the consequences might be, and whether she had other options. A large part of our initial goal setting was to improve her energy so she could tackle the lingering trauma of her birth experiences.

What the Testing Showed

Almost all of Jennifer's micronutrient levels were lower than normal. No wonder she was so exhausted and stressed!

Jennifer's Protocol

I gave Jennifer an intravenous solution of iron as well an oral iron supplement to help with her energy; DHA and DHEA to help improve mental clarity, cognitive function, and physical endurance; and an adaptogenic herb mix with ashwagandha and licorice. She did weekly sessions of restorative yoga, and for sleep she took melatonin and blocked out the blue light from her devices, which made a huge difference in both getting to sleep and staying asleep. She described her recovery as remarkable and then had the clarity and calmness to start seeing a therapist specializing in birth-trauma issues. The last time I needed to see her, she was six months pregnant, was feeling happy and full of vitality, and had a sense of well-being that she hadn't had with her previous pregnancies. In fact, she felt she had almost too much energy and was focusing on not getting too rushed and busy! Now that she had all the tools she needed to prevent depletion, I knew I wouldn't need to see her after this baby was born.

Generally, what I find is that mothers can feel trapped by the overwhelming feeling that their issues are too big to be improved by supplements and lifestyle interventions. I truly believe that micronutrient rebuilding can help mothers start to feel better physically and emotionally. You can also bring this book to your doctor if you want to have a conversation about what tests you'd like to get and what kinds of treatments are available to you. Once a mother's individual needs are identified, I see improvements happen quickly, and the ability to address the issues of powerlessness and overwhelm become easier as time goes on.

Step 1: Take these assessments to find potential deficiencies.

Step 2: See your doctor and ask for the recommended tests.

Blood tests should include iron studies, full blood count (CBC/FBC), electrolytes (EUC/BUN) including corrected calcium and liver function tests (LFT), thyroid blood tests including free T3, free T4, TSH, reverse T3, and thyroid antibodies, vitamin B_{12}, 25-OH vitamin D levels, plasma zinc, serum copper, ceruloplasmin, homocysteine, and whole blood histamine.

Urine tests should include morning spot iodine and twenty-four-hour urinary magnesium.

Saliva hormone testing should include melatonin x2, DHEAs x1, testosterone x1, cortisol x4, done at waking, 6 to 8 a.m.; 12 p.m.; 4 p.m.; or bedtime, 8 to 10 p.m.

Step 3: Work out a treatment plan with your provider, incorporating the supplements suggested in this book.

CHAPTER 5

Rebuilding Macronutrients

There is so much misinformation about the food we eat that it's almost impossible to know what to buy and how to cook. Every week, it seems, there's another miracle diet book or food fad or so-called expert telling us that what we thought was nutritious is actually harming us. What a lot of these fad-diet creators count on is the public's lack of understanding about both food and how bodies work. And because they tailor their findings to the general population, anyone suffering from postnatal depletion is automatically excluded.

This is truly a shame and in the end leaves people frustrated when they can't lose weight or feel better no matter how hard they try. It turns food into an adversary. Isn't that crazy? I love food. My patients love food. And we all love the saying "Food should be enjoyed, not endured." If your diet is nutritious but so restrictive and hard to follow that you feel like you're stuck enduring something miserable, all the good food in the world isn't going to make you feel better.

It's really hard to stick to a diet when you don't enjoy it. This is a key concept because the first step in undoing your postnatal depletion is, as you learned in the previous chapter, rebuilding your *micronutrients*. The second step is rebuilding your *macronutrients*. These are the proteins, carbohydrates, and fats you eat every day. You will not succeed in either of these steps if you're on a diet that makes you feel averse to what you're eating.

Pregnancy, childbirth, and breastfeeding put significantly more demands on our protein and fat metabolism than they do on our carbohydrate metabolism, but our fat-phobic Western society favors a diet that typically includes more carbohydrates than proteins and fat. Busy moms don't have time to surround themselves with healthy meals and snacks, and they often need to prepare meals that cater to the pickiest common denominator at the table rather than what's most nutritious. Hence, both societal diet norms and familial pressure foster the perfect conditions for macronutrient depletion.

The ideal diet for a woman recovering from depletion includes moderate to high levels of fat, moderate levels of protein, and small amounts of carbohydrates in her meals every day. Eating the right amounts of these macronutrients will make your repletion process so much easier and so much faster, and in this chapter I'll show you how to rethink the proportions of what you eat.

THE BEST FUEL FOR YOUR BODY

Your body is a "trifuel" vehicle: proteins, fats, and carbohydrates can all be transformed into the energy you need to stay alive. For most people, the body's preferred fuel is fat. Fat is like the nice thick log you put in the fireplace—the one that gives off steady and controlled warmth over a long period.

Carbohydrates, which your body transforms into sugars, are like the kindling you use to get your fire started. It quickly ignites, burns hot and fast, and then flames out. Remember the last time you got a sugar rush from eating a candy bar and then you were exhausted an hour later? That's what sugar does to you.

Protein is like a damp log that is hard to ignite, but if you persevere you can finally get it going. Your body can use protein for fuel, but only as a last resort, because getting energy out of it is a difficult process.

Chapter 9 covers my eating plan in detail, but for now read on so you can better understand why macronutrients have such a strong effect on your postnatal depletion.

WITH CALORIES, QUALITY, NOT QUANTITY, COUNTS

A calorie is a unit of energy and is measured in grams. One gram of fat contains 9 calories. One gram of protein or carbohydrates contains about 4 calories. An average adult woman needs approximately 1,800 calories each day to maintain her weight; an active woman needs an extra 200 to 400 calories. When you're pregnant, you need 200 to 300 additional calories every day, and when you're breastfeeding you need an extra 500 calories.

But here's where you need to be a calorie myth buster. The *quality* of calories is much more important than the *quantity* of calories you're eating. Your body doesn't process calories equally, so sticking to the equation of calories in/calories out is counterproductive. Eating 350 calories of candy is not the same as eating 350 calories of a chicken stir-fry with mixed vegetables—of course you know that! So instead of counting calories (and then beating yourself up emotionally when you miss your target), take into account how you're feeling and how strong your energy levels are. That's what really counts.

ABOUT FATS

It's unfortunate that the word *fat* covers the entire spectrum of good, healthy fats and bad ones that can harm you. Fats are the most important thing that we eat. Your brain is composed primarily of fat. You need fats for energy production and hormone production. Your skin needs a cushion of fat so you look good, too. In fact, every cell in our body is lined by a double layer of fat, which supports the cell's membrane. Fat is vital for life.

But just as calories differ in terms of quality, so, too, do fats. Comparing a good-quality fat like butter or ghee made from the milk of grass-fed cows to a bad fat like highly refined canola oil is like comparing diamonds with bricks and thinking that they're basically the same just because they're both rocks!

When I was working as a junior doctor in aboriginal health in northern Australia, I was amazed that the most prized foods in aboriginal culture tended to be the ones with the highest fat content, such as kangaroo tail, the fatty deposit within the goanna lizard, and specific cuts of turtle meat. I soon learned that among all indigenous cultures a pregnant woman's diet tended to be high in good-quality fats, whether from whale blubber harvested in the Aleutian Islands or butter made from the first spring grazing in the high parts of the Swiss Alps or certain types of fish eggs found in much of Asia. This is no accident. The societies that traditionally had access to high-quality fats tended to experience better health and better fertility.

Yet we live in a fat-phobic world. Our phobias are built on bogus scientific claims, a beauty aesthetic that overvalues a skinny frame, and a food industry that thrives on misperceptions. The sugar lobby did an excellent job at convincing the public that fat in food was bad. So what was all this fat replaced by? Sugar, of course—which made people gain even more weight. The food industry also uses fat phobia as a strategy to sell highly processed and nutrient-poor food—packaged junk food. In our local supermarket, I recently saw a bottle of golden syrup (which is similar to Karo syrup and is 100 percent sugar) that, in an extreme example of ludicrous food labeling, was advertised as cholesterol- and gluten-free! Clever food marketers capitalize on the fact that mothers who only want to do the best for themselves and their families are going to be more sensitive to advertising about health claims and body image, and this makes them particularly susceptible to advice, sales hooks, and food trends, whether good or bad.

The Fats You Need

What are fats, and how do you distinguish between the good and the bad ones? Here's a primer.

A fat is a chain of carbons (like a necklace) with a carboxylic acid at one end (like a clasp). The number of double bonds between the carbons in the fatty acid molecules determines whether a fat is saturated, monounsaturated, or polyunsaturated. Saturated fats have no double bonds between the carbons; unsaturated fats have at least one double bond (monounsaturated) or many double bonds (polyunsaturated).

Got that?

It is important to understand this information, because the double bonds in unsaturated fats are highly susceptible to oxidation or damage. Your body can still use these damaged fats for its needs, but you will pay the price for it. It is much better to use healthy fats rather than damaged ones when making the membranes of your cells. Given a chance, your body will replace these damaged fats with healthy ones. This is why choosing good unsaturated fats is so important, especially when you are pregnant or depleted.

You should always do your utmost to avoid bad fats that have been damaged or oxidized. Trans fats, for example, have been deliberately damaged to become more solid at room temperature. This is called hydrogenation, and it might be a good thing for industrial cookie and cake bakers, but it is definitely not good for you! Fortunately, trans fats are being phased out in the United States—you can see "No Trans Fats" food labels now. Unfortunately, in Australia no such legislation has been passed or is likely to be passed in the near future.

Other bad fats include any oils such as canola, soybean, cottonseed, sunflower, or peanut that are usually used in deep fryers or for battered food such as french fries and potato chips. These oils put you at risk for inflammation due to the way they are processed by your body; they make your white blood cells more reactive and pro-inflammatory while having a negative effect on both the health of your arteries and the quality of blood flow to your brain. I always advise mothers to remove these oils from the home and avoid them where possible when eating out. Replace them with coconut oil, olive oil, avocado oil, red palm oil, and solid animal fats such as butter, ghee, duck fat, tallow, or lard. Nut oils, such as walnut, macadamia, and almond, are also good. Just remember that peanuts are not nuts, so peanut oil should also be avoided.

An extremely important fat is omega-3 DHA. It's found primarily in fish, with lesser amounts in organ meats, egg yolks, and dairy fats such as ghee and butter (but not in whole milk). When you have postnatal depletion, replenishing this fat is crucial.

Omega-3 fatty acids from plant sources such as flaxseed can be converted in limited amounts into DHA by your body. But the more stressed and depleted your body is, the more inefficient and slow this conversion process to DHA becomes. You already learned in chapter 2 that a third of the dry weight of your brain is pure DHA, and you also know what happens to your DHA when you're pregnant if you don't get enough of it in your diet. There's basically a daylight robbery of DHA from your brain right into your developing baby's brain—and you pay the price! Low DHA in the brain and central nervous system directly contributes to both baby brain and postnatal anxiety.

Basically, the more omega-3s you have in your diet, the better you will feel. Strive to eat a 6-ounce piece of fish high in omega-3s three times per week as a baseline, which will typically give you around 1 g DHA per serving. Fish with high omega-3 levels that also have relatively low mercury levels are salmon, herring, mackerel (except for king mackerel), anchovies, bluefish, sardines, mullet, and lake trout. If you're not a fish lover, you can always take a supplement instead.

How to Treat DHA Deficiency

Because DHA deficiency is so common in depleted moms, I include DHA supplementation in almost all my protocols for my patients. The best source of DHA is fish oil; for vegetarians, it is algae oil.

It's important to know that fish can't make their own omega-3 fatty acids. They simply accumulate them, thanks to their diet, just as you accumulate fat-soluble vitamins from your diet. First, algae create the omega-3s DHA and EPA (eicosapentaenoic acid). Algae then get eaten by smaller marine animals such as crustaceans, which, in turn, get eaten by larger marine animals, and so on up the food chain. Unfortunately, because of our modern fishing practices and the pollution of our oceans, we might be nearing the end of fish-oil DHA production, and the best source of these precious omega-3s will be algae, not fish. This is why more and more people are turning to algae oil supplements for DHA.

ABOUT PROTEINS

The building blocks for your muscles and collagen, proteins are a vitally important component of your body. Collagen is what gives our skin and tissues elasticity and springiness and what gives our tendons and ligaments strength. Proteins are also involved in every aspect of cellular metabolism, especially as they are the essential part of making enzymes—and enzymes are the "get stuff done" machines inside your cells. Enzymes help you grow, rebuild and replace your tissues, detoxify and cleanse your body, and are responsible for all the housekeeping, too.

Proteins are made up of amino acids, which join together to form long chains called peptides. Amino acids are essential (your body can't make them, so they must come from food), nonessential (your body makes them), or conditional (you need them only when you're stressed or sick).

A complete protein (meat, poultry, dairy, seafood, eggs) has all of the nine essential amino acids in roughly the same amounts. An incomplete protein (beans, nuts, whole grains, seeds, corn) has only a few of the essential amino acids in significant amounts. You can combine two incomplete proteins and create a complete one. Plant proteins are not, in fact, incomplete, but they are *complementary* with other plant proteins. One good protein food added to another good protein food can make a great protein combination—rice and beans, quinoa and soy, and hummus and whole-grain pita are perfect examples. In my view, the most effective source of protein that helps speed up a mother's recovery is related to collagen, which comes from the ligaments and bones of animals. It's found in bone broths, in slow-cooked meats, and as a powdered supplement that can be added to soups and smoothies.

Calculating how much protein you need is not easy, because there are three parts to this equation: protein intake, protein absorption, and protein utilization. Protein intake is the amount and the quality of the protein you eat. Protein absorption relates to how efficiently our digestive system processes protein (and, yes, it starts with chewing!) and how well it gets absorbed into our bloodstream. Protein utilization is a little more complicated. On average only 50 percent of the protein you eat will make it into your bloodstream. The remaining 50 percent goes toward the creation and re-formation of the sausage-casing-like lining of your intestine. The good news is that despite protein deficiency's being very common postnatally, it doesn't take long to correct it.

How to Treat Protein Deficiency

Be warned that you will find much variation in the advice about your protein needs by different experts. When I create an individualized diet for a depleted mother, I usually prescribe a higher-fat, lower-carbohydrate diet with adequate protein. This is to correct the typical macronutrient imbalance that I see postnatally.

The average adult woman needs 45 to 60 g protein every day. When you're pregnant, you need an extra 10 g per day, and when you're breastfeeding you need an extra 20 g per day. There are nearly 50 g protein in an 8-ounce steak, so if you eat that and 2 cups Greek yogurt (19 g protein), you're close to the target.

When you are recovering from the birthing process, you will absolutely need more protein. Consider yourself like an athlete who was in training for the Olympics—you put an enormous strain on your body not only creating and birthing a child but also in the postdelivery repair of your uterus and birth canal. The protein drain continues if you're breastfeeding.

The nutritional rule of thumb is to incorporate a palm-size portion of high-protein food with each major meal, remembering to measure with your palm, not someone else's. This is typically a 2- to 3-ounce portion (and is a lot less than what you're used to seeing on your plate in a restaurant!).

You need to eat the best possible *kind* of protein. As with all food, quality is everything. Protein sources like legumes, fish, eggs, nuts, vegetables, dairy, and poultry are ideal. High-quality red meats are also good, in moderation. When your body is running well, you don't need a lot of red meat—maybe once or twice per week. It can be difficult to digest, and if you eat too much, it can contribute, I believe, to inflammation. When bodies are growing (such as children's or pregnant mothers') or are repairing and restoring (e.g., following birth or surgery or during breastfeeding, and/or in response to depletion), it's fine to eat red meat more frequently, as the benefits from its specific nutrients outweigh the inflammation that it may create. In these cases, I recommend eating 3 ounces red meat every other day during this time.

One of the best ways to give yourself predigested collagen is via bone broth. Simmering meat or poultry bones in water for many hours breaks down the collagen—you'll know when this happens if your broth becomes like Jell-O after you leave it in the fridge overnight. Many indigenous cultures, as you read earlier in the book, use slow-cooked bone broths as nourishing meals for new mothers, and they're incredibly easy to make or buy.

If you're using supplements to boost the protein content of your diet, it's important to choose carefully. I don't recommend whey-based protein shakes and bars because I find that they seem to add to inflammation, not improve it, in a significant proportion of my patients. Instead, look for high-quality plant-based protein powders (such as hemp seed or brown rice protein powder) and high-quality denatured collagen powders as simple add-ons to your regular diet, especially during the restoration process and for those days when you don't have time to cook. Adding these powders to smoothies or soups is a popular option.

How to Treat Amino Acid Deficiency

Occasionally, specific amino acid deficiencies, which are not necessarily caused by pregnancy, can also affect and enhance your depletion. Although they are not straightforward to diagnose, the best test to ask for is a urinary amino acid test. I tend to request this test only if a mother has severe lethargy or severe mental health issues, such as debilitating anxiety.

We know that stress can deplete certain amino acids. When the hormone cortisol is released by your adrenal gland in response to stress, this can decrease your levels of the essential amino acid tryptophan and is a contributing factor to the severity of postnatal anxiety and depression. The supplement I use to treat this is 5-HTP (5-hydroxytryptophan), a modified type of tryptophan; a typical dose is between 50 and 300 mg daily. (This cannot be taken if you are on antidepressants.)

In addition, deficiency in certain micronutrients can also negatively affect your amino acids, particularly lysine and methionine. You need those two amino acids in order to create the energy-producing molecule carnitine—but this process requires iron and vitamins B_3, B_6, and C.

Insufficiencies and deficiencies can compound and exacerbate your postnatal depletion, but starting small with the repletion of micronutrients will make it easier to rebuild your macronutrients, too. These examples show the intricate balancing act that nutrients perform with one another. With the right supplements and dietary and behavioral adjustments, restoring equilibrium can be a straightforward task.

ABOUT CARBOHYDRATES

When you're depleted, the last thing you should look at is the food pyramid of the Western diet that was used for many years—the one that taught us that carbs are the main source of energy. Couple that with a food industry that sells "healthy" packaged and processed food to millions of people, and you have a guaranteed recipe for weight gain, health issues, and an inability to manage your postnatal depletion. I often joke with my patients about "cardboard-hydrates." Not all carbs are bad, but increasingly the nutritional profile of the ingredients making it into our food isn't much different from the cardboard box itself!

Carbohydrates are basically chains of saccharide (or sugar) molecules.

Short chains are the simple sugars and tend to be sweet (sugar, dairy, processed grains, and fruit). Longer chains are the complex carbohydrates (whole grains, green vegetables, legumes, beans, peanuts, potatoes, and corn). Simple carbs are quickly digested, while complex carbs usually contain a lot of fiber that slows down the digestive process and makes you feel fuller for longer while also providing food in the form of prebiotics for your beneficial gut flora.

Whenever you eat carbs, your body has to break them down into the basic sugar molecules (usually glucose) so that they can then be transported around the body. There is usually the equivalent of 1 teaspoon sugar floating around in your bloodstream at any given time.

Normally, thanks to the hormone you know as insulin, your body is extremely good at keeping your blood sugar at a very stable level. Your pancreas, sensing the incoming sugar from your digestive tract, releases very small amounts of insulin to escort these sugars into your cells and liver. With complex carbs, the sugars are released gradually into the bloodstream and the insulin system manages this easily.

Not so with simple sugars. If you drink a can of soda, which contains up to 12 teaspoons sugar, you've just ingested twelve times the amount of sugar that is already circulating in your bloodstream. Your pancreas does the equivalent of a freak-out as it struggles to cope with this sudden influx of sugar, and it releases much more insulin than you'd normally need. This is what causes a sugar, or energy, rush (lots of insulin dealing with your blood sugar as it gets stored), followed by a crash (your blood sugar wobbling as your insulin rapidly returns to baseline, leaving you tired, shaky, or foggy), then followed by even more insatiable cravings for sugar (your brain, not able to figure out where all the sugar went, telling you it wants more, more, more!). Over time, this vicious cycle of sugar cravings followed by energy spikes, fatigue, and more cravings leads to insulin resistance, which is the precursor to metabolic syndrome and type 2 diabetes, a serious, life-threatening disease.

In addition, when you burn primarily sugar, your stress systems will become more hyperactive, and it will take fewer stimuli for you to become stressed. It also becomes harder for your body to return to its baseline weight and manage inflammation when you are burning primarily sugar or when your excess sugar isn't burned off but instead is stored as fat. Turning to low-fat or fat-free foods, which substitute sugar for fat, is not the answer. Consuming sugar-laden foods will not help anyone lose weight. It's one of the reasons why so many diets fail.

The Carbohydrates You Need

As discussed earlier, the quality of your calories is much more important than the quantity, and the quality of your carbohydrates is no exception. The average adult woman needs to eat approximately 150 g carbs every day. When you are pregnant, you should eat 175 g, and when you are breastfeeding you should eat 210 g. Keep in mind that these figures are approximations and may fluctuate when variables like height, weight, and age are factored in. There is also ongoing debate about these figures in the medical and nutrition fields; a recent study from the Commonwealth Scientific and Industrial Research Organization in Australia showed that a low-carbohydrate diet of 50 to 75 g daily is helpful for people with metabolic syndrome and diabetes, especially in improving and in many cases reversing their diabetes.

In my experience, women with postnatal depletion respond best to a low- or no-grain diet until they are feeling much improved in their energy and overall sense of well-being. This short-term diet tends to be less inflammatory, is more nutrient dense, and eventually leads to more stable blood sugars. Most of the carbohydrates you do eat should come from fresh colorful vegetables—the brighter the color, the more nutrients the food contains.

You'll see what to eat in chapter 9, and there will be meal plans to help you. I promise you that you won't be hungry!

How to Treat Carbohydrate Deficiency

Because the typical American diet is carbohydrate based, it is extremely rare to find carbohydrate deficiencies. Bear in mind, however, that while eating junk carbs made with processed flour and white sugar will give you an excess of carbohydrates, it also means you aren't getting the good nutrients you need. I tend to talk to patients about the king of the carbs being aboveground vegetables, including the cruciferous veggies cabbage and broccoli or vegetables from the allium family such as leeks and onions. The okay carbs in moderation include belowground vegetables, fruit, legumes, beans, and basmati/brown rice. The bad carbs tend to be all-white, processed, and packaged. Think fresh and green and you can't go wrong.

CHAPTER 6

Rebuilding Hormones

A creaky old saying that I first heard in medical school when learning about hormones was that women have "her-moans" and men have "his-moans." What I discovered since is that women tend to have a very intricate up-and-down orchestration of their hormones, and while men tend to have much more consistency with theirs, as a man's hormones gradually decline over his lifetime, leading to what's often described as grumpy old man syndrome—hence, "his-moans." (Told you it was creaky—don't shoot the messenger!)

Hormones might have borne the brunt of this creakiness, but to tell you the truth, I find them to be the least understood part of how our bodies work while being one of the most important. And when your hormones are all over the place and you are depleted and feel terrible, *you* have a legitimate reason to moan!

A HORMONE PRIMER

What are hormones? According to the dictionary, a hormone is a "chemical substance produced in the body that controls and regulates the activity of certain cells or organs." Basically, a hormone is a signal or a messenger that moves from one part of your body to another, barking out orders so everything works as it's meant to.

Hormones are produced in different glands in your body. They are regulated by the section of the brain called the hypothalamus, which sends signals to your pituitary gland, also found in the brain, which, in turn, sends out signals to the hormone-producing glands. The hormones that have a direct effect on your postnatal depletion are the thyroid hormones, the adrenal hormones (cortisol and DHEA), melatonin, and the ovarian hormones (estrogen and progesterone). Each hormone has a specific function.

When you're healthy, hormones are released by your various glands and scurry around your bloodstream, telling your organs what and how much to do. But when you're depleted, these hormonal signals can get out of whack, resulting in too many or too few hormones being released.

For example, if you are on a nutrient-poor fat-free diet because you want to lose baby weight, this type of diet is likely to send signals to your brain that a strange type of famine is taking place. Your body reacts by going into starvation mode, and signals are sent to slow down your metabolism. This, of course, makes you need even fewer calories, so you *gain* weight even if you aren't eating very much. (This is one of the reasons calorie-restrictive diets just don't work over the long term.)

What Happens to Your Hormones When You're Pregnant

When you're pregnant, there is a tremendous hormonal surge: essentially all the symptoms of pregnancy are related to estrogen (causing a lot of the swelling and loosening of body tissue, possibly resulting in acid reflux, hemorrhoids, constipation, varicose veins, and lethargy) and progesterone (which can add to the elation of pregnancy, though one in ten women experiences depression during pregnancy).

- Estrogen increases to up to *thirty times* your prepregnancy levels, as it's needed for uterus and breast enlargement as well for increasing your body fluids. (Half of this estrogen increase is made by the mother, and the other half is made by the placenta.)
- Progesterone increases to ten times your prepregnancy levels in the last trimester, stimulating placental growth and allowing maturation of your breast tissue to get you ready for milk

production. Progesterone is what causes the relaxed feelings of well-being that many mothers experience during pregnancy.

- Thyroid hormone production increases 50 percent by the third trimester, allowing for proper growth of the developing fetus's brain as well as meeting the thyroid needs of the mother.
- Cortisol production is controlled for most of the pregnancy by the mother, but in the last trimester that control switches over to the placenta; cortisol production increases to three times your prepregnancy levels. It is likely that the baby, via the placenta, is trying to keep the mother healthy, alert, and energized. This cortisol boost can manifest in a number of ways; you may find yourself stepping up your activity level, perhaps wanting to get the nursery ready for painting or clearing out the garage. It can also contribute to irritability, anxiety, and a feeling of "I just want this thing out of me now and I can't wait for this pregnancy to be over!"

After the delivery of the placenta, your estrogen levels will drop a whopping 90 to 95 percent, while your progesterone levels will drop to nearly zero within the forty-eight hours after birth. The levels of CRH (corticotropin-releasing hormone), a brain hormone that facilitates cortisol production in your system, will also plummet, and if you are not physically and emotionally nurtured in the early weeks after delivery, then your CRH levels will *not* return to normal levels. Low cortisol contributes to lethargy and a sense of inertia and is also associated with allergy flare-ups; it is even thought to contribute to the progression of postpartum autoimmune disease.

If you are breastfeeding, then your levels of estrogen and progesterone are suppressed, and your period should not start up again. But if you have low estrogen and progesterone combined with low cortisol, low DHEA (which is typically seen postpartum), and thyroid hormone imbalances, you may feel like you've been in a car crash. If you're also sleep deprived, you'll become further depleted.

I believe this is why mothers need to have at least a *month* of the kind of fully supported recovery we see in the many cultures I wrote about in chapter 1. This care and nurturing gives mothers the time they need for their hormone systems to reset.

HAVE YOUR HORMONES CHECKED!

Aside from estrogen and progesterone, hormonal levels are often ignored or downplayed in mothers who have postnatal depletion. Can you believe it? I'll bet you can. It is one of the simplest things to check, yet it's overlooked so often that I get incredibly frustrated on behalf of my patients. So it's absolutely essential for you to know what low hormonal levels can do to you so you can address any imbalances.

I've found that for those having hormonal problems, and especially women with postnatal depletion, the knee-jerk reaction by mainstream medicine is to give more hormones. While this may have some short-term benefits, it doesn't address the cause and can actually make it more difficult to treat any underlying issues.

Make Lifestyle Changes *First*

To fix hormone depletion, you must start with lifestyle modifications. This means getting enough sleep and getting enough rest. You also need to improve your diet, move more, and do your best to get some downtime so that you can relax. Now, before you throw the book against the wall, I'm not suggesting that eight hours of uninterrupted sleep, hours of yoga and meditation per day, and three perfectly balanced, healthy meals per day is the only way to restore healthy hormone levels. One of the reasons that postnatal depletion is so pernicious is that it flares up just as you enter a phase of life that is likely more taxing physically and emotionally than anything you've experienced before. So how can you practice this all-important self-care given such challenging circumstances?

One of the hardest things for mothers to do is embrace the change in priorities and abilities that comes with having children. It can be a shock to find that your sleep is not your own, your time is not your own, and your space is not your own. How many mothers know the pain of a bursting bladder or pins and needles in their arm yet tolerate it so as not to wake the baby? Figuring out a way to incorporate the things you loved before your child was born into your new life as a parent can feel like reinventing the wheel. It's a whole new world of responsibilities and needs, and it's easy to become so focused on your child that you lose sight of yourself. But it's crucial that you take care of yourself and ask for as much help as you need, because restoring your body is the first step in feeling like yourself again.

What I'd like you to do is play first and work later. In other words, now that you have a child, bring that magical child's sense of wonder into your own life. This isn't about surrendering to escapism but surrendering to *play*. You do this by incorporating song, music, dance, silliness, and laughter as much as you possibly can. There will always be work, chores, and responsibilities, and it can be frustrating to see those duties unattended. But make sure that you also allow yourself some time to enjoy your family, even if that sometimes means going through your to-do list a little slower than you would like.

This is not a request for you to lower your standards. There is a real benefit to taking some time for deliberate play. Adding playtime into your life is guaranteed to help lower your stress levels—and you know by now how important it is that your stress levels stay as low as possible. This is where support from your family and friends is so important, too. Having people help you with the cleaning and laundry and food shopping and meal preparation can make all the difference in your stress levels. I see so many depleted mothers using precious energy on entertaining well-meaning visitors who just want to coo over the baby. That is totally understandable, of course, but it means you're usually the one who's paying the price for those visits! When guests want to visit, find ways to ask them for help, whether it's bringing over a meal or doing some laundry. If you don't feel comfortable putting your guests to work, carve out a little time for yourself while you have the extra hands! While they are holding the baby, you can take a shower, do a little movement—or take a nap!

If one of my patients finds that making these lifestyle modifications doesn't help, or if her need for repletion and recovery is more immediate, then I'll often prescribe the bioactive form of female hormones to get her body back in sync. Bioactives are hormones that occur in nature (usually found in plants or animal tissue) and are identical to what the body produces, so your body will easily recognize them and know how to utilize and metabolize them. I've found that they work better for my patients than synthetic hormones do. (Discuss this option with your gynecologist.) Bioactive hormones will often be used in combination with herbs and the other measures mentioned in the book.

A GUIDE TO YOUR HORMONES

T3 and T4—Your Thyroid Hormones

The thyroid is a small gland in your neck that regulates your metabolism. Your pituitary gland sends TSH (thyroid-stimulating hormone) to the thyroid to produce its hormones T4 and T3. T4 is inactive, and acts as a sort of reservoir for your body to then convert to T3, which is the active hormone. Along with cortisol (the stress hormone, which you'll read about in the next section), T3 then tells your cells how much energy to make. If your thyroid is overactive, this is called *hyper*thyroidism, and it can cause rapid or irregular heartbeat; nervousness, irritability, and mood swings; weight loss; heat intolerance; fatigue and sleep problems; hand tremors; muscle weakness and palpitations; and goiters (an enlarged thyroid that causes your neck to swell and your eyes to bulge outward). When you don't have enough thyroid hormones, it's called *hypo*thyroidism, and it can cause weight gain; depression; a slowed heart rate; dry skin, hair, and nails; insomnia; constipation; irregularities with your menstrual cycle as well as infertility; and a sensitivity to cold. Having an underactive thyroid will greatly slow down your recovery time and can become a major issue in itself, not just a contributing factor to postnatal depletion.

How to Test for T3 and T4 Levels

Measuring TSH, T3, and T4 levels in a blood test will tell you about your thyroid's health. You may also need blood tests for thyroid antibodies and an ultrasound of your thyroid if there is any question of swelling in your neck or enlargement of the thyroid gland.

A useful addition to blood work is to measure your body's basal temperature as soon as you wake up for at least two weeks. The reason this is helpful is because heat is a measure of how much activity/energy your body is producing. (People with low thyroid hormones often feel cold, and this is one of the reasons why.) Monitoring thyroid function with both blood tests and basal body temperatures is very important, yet it is often not recommended or is overlooked. If your average temperature is approaching 98.6°F and your TSH is close to the ideal range of 1 to 2 mIU/L, then a thyroid problem is unlikely. If, however, your temperature is consistently below 97.8°F and your TSH is above 3 mIU/L, hypothyroidism is very likely. If you are concerned, talk to your doctor and request a TSH test and, if possible, a free T3 and free T4 test, too.

How to Treat Thyroid Hormone Deficiencies

If you have hyperthyroidism (usually in the form of the autoimmune conditions of postpartum thyroiditis or Graves' disease), then your doctor will prescribe antithyroid or beta-blocking medications.

If you have hypothyroidism (usually in the form of the autoimmune conditions of postpartum thyroiditis or Hashimoto's disease, or from low iodine or tyrosine levels), then you will normally start with a more conservative approach of replacing tyrosine (in pill form) and iodine (via drops or a sublingual spray) if levels are low. Supporting recovery via sleep will also help. Thyroid function needs to be rechecked frequently—usually every four weeks—and if there is little improvement, then a thyroid hormone supplement can be used. These are not a sentence for life, and once the levels are back on track I can usually wean mothers off them. If, however, you have had significant thyroid inflammation and/or damage to the thyroid tissue, which are checked via blood tests, then you might need to go on supplements long-term.

There are four options for thyroid supplementation: levothyroxine (synthetic T4), thyroid extract (a combination of T4/T3), slow-release T3, and Liotrix (synthetic T4/T3). I tend to recommend the first two, but one option is not necessarily superior to the others. What's most important is that you're monitored long-term every three to six months by a practitioner who has experience in thyroid supplementation. This is essential not just for your own sense of well-being but to ensure that your treatment is correct.

Cortisol—Your Adrenal Hormone

Cortisol is the main hormone produced in the adrenal glands, located on top of your kidneys. It is essential for energy regulation in your body and is released in response to stress. Remember that normal body stress is not always *bad* stress. You experience normal body stress when you engage in basic activities like exercise or making love. You experience normal stress when it's time to get up in the morning: like a good drill sergeant, your cortisol (which peaks around 8:00 or 9:00 a.m.) gets you up and dressed, prepares you to get the baby up and fed—and then pushes you to get dressed again after baby's breakfast ends up on your first set of clothes!

Cortisol release becomes a problem when too many demands are put on your body at once. An instant release of cortisol will help you navigate a situation in which you're driving with the baby in the back, a car runs through a stop sign, and you swerve to avoid it. Everything is fine, and you take some deep breaths, put on some soothing music, glance back at your sweetly sleeping baby, and drive off calmly. But if the baby suddenly wakes up and starts screaming and you realize you haven't eaten yet and you get stuck in traffic and you're late for day care and work, too, and then a red light goes on in your car, your cortisol levels are going to skyrocket. This is one of the reasons you might find it hard to lose the belly fat after your baby is born—prolonged high cortisol levels increase other hormone levels, which tell your body to *hold on* to this fat and keep you in sugar-burning mode. How fair is that? Not fair at all!

If these problems multiply over the course of the day, your body is going to let you know. You will get cortisol fluctuations when you are hungry or tired (what is called "hangry"). Unfortunately, this often happens at night when your exhausted body is trying to sleep. These cortisol spikes can lead to flushes and surges and leave you feeling panicked and anxious. The state is sometimes referred to as tired and wired.

Cortisol is just not intended to be on high alert all the time. After a while—and this often takes years of ongoing and unrelenting stress to occur—your body basically gets pissed off and your brain sends out a signal to lower cortisol production levels. It's as if your brain is like the accelerator and the adrenals are like the engine in your car. The engine is fine, but the accelerator pedal is stuck at one low speed. No matter how much you pump it, you can't get the car to go the way it should. This is how my depleted patients experience adrenal fatigue—they're running on empty.

How to Test for Cortisol Levels

The simplest and most accurate measurement is via saliva hormone testing. Ask your doctor or naturopath for a test kit, where at home you put saliva into vials at four different times during the day, typically at 8 a.m., 12 p.m., 4 p.m., and 8 p.m., and then send them off to a lab.

How to Treat Cortisol Deficiencies and Excess

Not surprisingly, the number one way to help restore cortisol levels is through sleep. It's the most important restorative activity you can do, along with weekly sessions of restorative yoga and/or restorative acupuncture.

I often also prescribe a regimen combining adrenal-supporting herbs with vitamin C (2 to 4 g per day) for six weeks, followed by either review or retesting. These herbs have been shown to help our resilience and ability to cope with stress and have been used by different cultures for thousands of years. My preferred herbs, due to both effectiveness and safety during pregnancy and breastfeeding, include ashwagandha (1 g twice per day) and rhodiola (100 mg twice per day).

If a mother remains fatigued, with very low cortisol and ACTH (adrenocorticotropic hormone) levels, and she hasn't responded to the initial treatments, then cortisol can be prescribed at low doses. As a short-term therapy for six to twelve weeks, it is both safe and effective for nursing mothers, with a dosage of 4 mg at 8 a.m. and 4 mg at 12 p.m. I would *not* recommend using higher doses, because this can lead to your body switching off its own cortisol production—the opposite of what we're trying to achieve!

If your cortisol levels are too high, you can also try the nonessential amino acid phosphatidyl serine, 200 mg twice per day for six weeks, and then retest. In this form, serine helps regulate levels postnatally. You would need to have your levels retested before having another course of serine.

You can also read about many different ways to reduce your stress/cortisol levels and rebuild your energy in the next chapter.

Estrogen and Progesterone—Your Ovaries' Hormones

There are three sex hormones produced by your ovaries: the female hormones estrogen and progesterone and, in small amounts, the male hormone testosterone. You need testosterone to maintain bone density, keep your skin supple, and support a healthy muscle-to-fat ratio in your body. Testosterone also has powerful antiaging effects, and it helps improve mood, stress resilience, and cognitive function.

Estrogen and progesterone are an awesome team and regulate your reproduction functions and fertility. After an egg is produced in your ovaries every month, estrogen and progesterone cause your uterine lining to thicken and mature; if the egg is not fertilized, you shed this lining when you get your period. If the egg is fertilized, enormous levels of estrogen and progesterone plus hCG (human chorionic gonadotropin) are released to stop other eggs from developing and to allow your pregnancy to proceed normally.

After your baby is born, your estrogen and progesterone levels plummet, as mentioned earlier. Usually, they won't go back to normal levels until your period resumes. The loss of the sense of well-being that estrogen and progesterone provide can be made up for via prolactin and oxytocin, two of the main hormones involved in breastfeeding and skin-to-skin contact. But it isn't always, and that can be a major contributor to the baby blues. If your other hormones don't return to optimal levels, you'll feel lethargic and anxious and find it hard to maintain a sense of well-being.

Even when your period resumes, there can still be problems. The roles of estrogen and progesterone are easily hijacked through stress, which causes a mismatch between their levels and effects. This mismatch is often what is responsible for the varying and sometimes quite different symptoms of a woman's newly established menstrual cycle, including shorter or longer cycle length, pelvic and abdominal pain, changes in menstrual blood flow, and duration of blood flow, as well as many psychological symptoms. In fact, many of the symptoms attributed to PMS (premenstrual syndrome) are caused and exacerbated by this mismatch. If you find yourself having PMS problems, be sure to discuss them with your health-care practitioner.

How to Test for Estrogen and Progesterone Levels

The ideal test for measuring ovarian hormones is saliva hormone testing, done halfway between ovulation and the first day of the menstrual bleeding. This is usually on day 21 of your monthly cycle, the point at which your estrogen and progesterone levels are both naturally at their highest. This will give you the most accurate information about not only your hormonal levels but also the interplay between progesterone and estrogen.

There is also a newer test that your health-care practitioner may request, the urinary steroid hormone test, which is helpful if you have an erratic monthly cycle or hard-to-diagnose hormonal issues. It maps your hormone levels and can be done on various days of your cycle, depending on the exact nature of the information required.

How to Treat Estrogen and Progesterone Excess and Deficiencies

Estrogen

Whether high or low, estrogen can have overlapping symptoms such as fatigue, insomnia, anxiety, depression, low libido, and mood swings with menstruation. Low estrogen is generally associated with dry skin, vaginal dryness, urinary tract infections, hot flashes, and night sweats, whereas high estrogen is associated with water retention and bloating, fibrocystic breast tissue, and fibroids.

Estrogen excess is more common than estrogen deficiency. Treatment for estrogen excess is with supplements that assist with its correct metabolism. These typically include extracts from cruciferous vegetables such as broccoli seed or celery, or from plants like flax. Your practitioner may prescribe supplements such as DIM (diindolylmethane, a phytochemical found in cruciferous vegetables), 200 to 400 mg daily, or calcium D glucurate, 1,500 to 3,000 mg daily.

If you are estrogen deficient, short-term support with low-dose estrogen creams is recommended. Estriol is the mildest and safest form, with a dose typically of 2 to 4 mg daily. Once menstruating estrogen levels are restored, estriol is usually no longer needed.

All supplementation must be done in conjunction with a health-care practitioner, and check-ins every six weeks are required until your hormones are rebalanced. Benefits from medication can take two weeks to appear, and monitoring and follow-up are crucial to ensure safety both postnatally (if you are breastfeeding) and in the long term.

Progesterone

Whether high or low, progesterone contributes to the symptoms of breast swelling. Low progesterone is associated with anxiety, mood swings, insomnia, low libido, fluid retention, endometriosis, cramping, PMS, and acne, whereas high progesterone is associated with gastrointestinal bloating and insulin resistance.

Progesterone, if abnormal, tends to be low, and my treatment starts with supplements of chaste tree/perilla/parsley leaf extract and quercetin. These need to be taken in conjunction with an experienced healthcare professional with retesting every six weeks. It usually takes about three to six months to feel better.

If higher levels are needed, I mainly use a transdermal progesterone cream, 10 to 15 mg daily. If you're menstruating, progesterone is used for only the last two weeks of your cycle. If you're not menstruating, then progesterone is typically used for three weeks of the month with a one-week break to help avoid progesterone resistance. Again, see your healthcare practitioner for follow-up every six weeks until your levels are back to normal.

If your progesterone is high, I would discuss this with your healthcare practitioner, as it is not a common part of postnatal depletion.

AMANDA'S REGIMEN

Amanda was thirty-six, with a two-year-old and a four-month-old baby. She was feeling sluggish and had no energy, had lost her motivation and vitality, was sleeping poorly, and felt that her brain "had gone on holiday." She'd also started to develop muscular aches and pains and was gaining weight. She was running an online business, which she described as stressful and causing her to have a short fuse.

What the Testing Showed

Amanda had low thyroid function (high TSH), low cortisol, low homocysteine, and low-normal vitamin D and DHEA.

Amanda's Protocol

Amanda was initially hesitant to start on anything artificial, including thyroid supplements, so I prescribed a regimen with adrenal and many different thyroid-supporting herbs to improve her energy and NAC to raise her homocysteine; in addition, I prescribed vitamin D supplements, which, along with NAC, would reduce inflammation and improve her cognition and sense of vitality. To improve her sleep, I advised her to allocate specific blocks of time for her business and to avoid computer use after 8:00 p.m.

After six weeks, Amanda was feeling and sleeping better, but many of her initial symptoms remained. Blood retests showed her that her thyroid function was still too low, so she started on levothyroxine (synthetic T4). This made all the difference, especially in terms of her weight and her "brain holiday."

I now see Amanda every six months to recheck her thyroid levels. She's feeling great and is thrilled that she can get enough sleep, have her old energy back, and manage her business.

ISABELLE'S REGIMEN

Isabelle was thirty-five, with an eighteen-month-old, whom she was still breastfeeding, and a three-year-old. She'd been diagnosed with Hashimoto's disease following the birth of her first child but had been put on an inadequate dose of thyroid medication with not much follow-up. As a result of this improper treatment, her hair was falling out (this is not an uncommon postnatal symptom, but in Isabelle's case her depletion was not the primary cause). She was also lethargic; she had abdominal bloating, forehead acne, which she'd never had before, and multiple chemical sensitivities; and she told me she felt like Led Zeppelin's "dazed and confused." She had trouble falling asleep yet woke up daily at 4:30 a.m. When asked about her libido, she laughed and said that the scoring system didn't go low enough to reflect her lack of sexual desire. She obviously retained her sense of humor but admitted she felt she was literally falling apart.

What the Testing Showed

Isabelle's thyroid hormones were very low, along with her iodine, iron, and vitamin D. Her pyrrole level was very high, which suggests high amounts of zinc loss in her urine, and she had an intestinal parasite. I explained to her that even though these issues are not typical of postnatal depletion per se, they are common postnatal occurrences. Isabelle was also sensitive to cow-based dairy protein and several grains and legumes.

Isabelle's Protocol

I immediately upped Isabelle's thyroid supplement and gave her an infusion of iron. She also took herbs for her parasite, a DHA supplement, micronutrients with zinc and vitamin D, and trace elements for her pyrrole disorder. A Paleo-type diet with a very low grain and legume intake for the initial three months was also suggested, and she was able to eat non-cow-based dairy. I also added a protein powder with mitochondrial nutrients, DHEA, and rhodiola.

Isabelle struggled with her diet at first, but she realized that all the elements of her protocol were important, and as her energy improved, she found it easier to manage her diet. After three months, she was greatly improved, but she needed to continue the regime for a further three months to really help her baby brain go away for good. As she began feeling better (and better about herself), her libido returned to normal, too. No more Led Zeppelin!

CHAPTER 7

Rebuilding Energy

When you're depleted, getting up to feed the baby can feel as difficult as it would to finish the last few miles of a marathon—you're that exhausted.

All the energy-building techniques described in this chapter build on the postnatal-repletion foundation that was laid out in previous chapters. After treating countless mothers with postnatal depletion, I've found that restorative therapies are amazingly beneficial for speeding up the recovery process.

Treatments can include acupuncture, Ayurvedic therapies, restorative yoga, mindfulness meditation, biofeedback such as HeartMath, and relaxation techniques, all of which can improve your energy when you use them strategically. Combine them with the get-better-sleep strategies in the next chapter as well as the gentle forms of exercise I suggest in chapter 10, and your foundation will grow ever stronger. Even if you want to try only one of these strategies at first, once you feel its effects you'll want to try more! They're great not just for specifically rebuilding your energy but also for generally improving all aspects of your health and well-being.

TRADITIONAL CHINESE MEDICINE, *JING* REPLETION, AND ACUPUNCTURE

For those of you who aren't familiar with the three Taoist treasures *qi* (or *chi*), *jing*, and *shen*, here's the gist:

- *Qi* is your life force and describes how strong your energy is at any given moment.
- *Jing* is your core, the primordial energy you were born with.
- *Shen* is your spiritual energy.

Think of these three treasures this way: *qi* is the flame of a candle, *jing* is the candle wax, and *shen* is the light from the candle being dispersed around the room.

In traditional Chinese medicine (TCM), *jing* depletion is what causes the aging process. It affects how you sleep and predisposes you to premature aging. (Take a look at how recent American presidents have aged in office, and you have tangible proof of what an accelerated *jing* depletion can do to someone.) Practices such as *qigong* and *tai chi*, along with acupuncture therapy and ingesting herbal teas and supplements, are designed to slowly regenerate *jing*.

Pregnancy and childbirth also cause what TCM practitioners call profound *qi* and blood deficiency. Breastfeeding, cold invasion (a TCM term for what happens when someone gets too cold), and blood stasis (sluggish circulation) make it even worse. According to TCM, if a recovering mother gets physically cold and does not receive the correct care or food during this vulnerable time, then she may enter into this profound state of *qi* and blood deficiency.

Jing depletion is harder to describe because we don't have a Western equivalent of this condition. Mothers with this deep depletion of core energy are beyond tired and will sometimes describe themselves as being utterly wiped out or burned-out or, as we say in Australia, "totally knackered." They don't even have the energy to say how little energy they have.

Obviously, everybody's energy-depletion levels are different and can vary from day to day. But because the concept of *jing* depletion is so foreign to Western medicine and our way of thinking, it is hard to get good advice on what to do about it or even to get sympathy from loved ones. I can't tell you how many moms have sat crying in my office, telling me that they are completely burned-out and desperate, yet the advice they've received consists only of platitudes: "Well, it sounds like you need some time out" or "Maybe you should go on a vacation and recover." For a depleted mom, with each day blurring into the next and no end in sight of the 24/7 child-care routine, that advice is not very useful!

It's far better to hear "You know what? I totally understand how exhausted you are. Your fatigue and lack of energy are very real and very debilitating, and I know you want to get your life back. Let's devise a plan together that will end your depletion and make you feel like yourself again—only better. I'm going to give you some information on some wonderful healing methods that will address this situation right away."

Traditional holistic treatments like acupuncture and Ayurvedic medicine have been used for thousands of years because they are effective and safe. It is hugely unfortunate that they are still considered "alternative" treatments, because they contain great wisdom and can make such an enormous difference in your health and healing. So, go for it!

About Acupuncture

Acupuncture has been used for more than five thousand years to treat all sorts of ailments. It is highly effective at helping your body heal, improving energy and stamina, fighting off viruses and infections, and managing pain. The basic premise behind it is that your body's *qi* travels around on certain meridians, and when these meridians become blocked your energy becomes blocked, too. Stimulating certain points with the insertion of microfine needles will allow the *qi* to flow smoothly again.

A body depleted of nutrients, blood, sleep, and exercise becomes disorganized and inefficient. The energy boost you feel after acupuncture treatment is not like what you get from coffee or stimulants; it comes about when your body and its organ systems can communicate better. Typically, the benefits from acupuncture last only one or two days at first, but with progressive treatments the benefits can easily last two to three weeks.

I've seen regular acupuncture sessions cut a new mom's depletion-recovery time from the typical six to nine months down to three months. Acupuncture's effects can be astonishingly effective for depletion, and many mainstream health-care practitioners now routinely prescribe acupuncture sessions as a welcome addition and enhancer to their more conventional treatments. Unless you have a needle phobia, there is absolutely no downside to acupuncture.

I urge you to find a licensed acupuncturist in your area. Many of them are also trained in the use of Chinese herbs in conjunction with the treatments, which can further speed up your repletion process.

AYURVEDA: THE INDIAN SYSTEM OF MEDICINE

Ayurveda is an ancient system of healing. It was first developed in India more than five thousand years ago and is based on the concept that every person comprises one of three fundamental energies, or *doshas*: *vata* (wind), *pitta* (fire), and *kapha* (earth). When a *dosha* is out of balance, Ayurveda treats it with a combination of diet, exercise, supplements, and stress-reduction techniques to bring the *dosha* back into balance.

Particularly important is what and how you eat, as Ayurveda believes that your *dosha* can be rebalanced when you eat foods in certain combinations. Foods are divided by six tastes—sweet, sour, salty, pungent, bitter, and astringent—with specific attributes for each one. Knowing this might explain why you tend to like certain tastes or have particular cravings; some people naturally gravitate to sour, like pickles, while others have a sweet tooth. Personally, I like salty the best. With the incredible range of herbs, spices, and food combinations within the Ayurvedic cooking tradition, these tastes can be used to help reset and rebalance any particular *dosha* that may be out of balance.

If you decide to try Ayurvedic treatments, find a highly skilled practitioner. The Ayurvedic system understands each person's constitution, so its tailored regimens can often work quickly to help with your energy, mental clarity, and motivation. I've seen how the combination of Ayurvedic herbs and supplements along with a custom-tailored diet can work wonders, but it's not something you can self-diagnose and treat.

AYURVEDA AND NEW MOTHERS

A new mom in the Ayurvedic tradition is called the *prasuta*, and there is a special period of recovery called the *sutika* that lasts for at least forty-two days.

The *prasuta* is in a delicate state during which imbalance of the *vata* is likely to occur, leading to anxiety, insecurity, dryness, digestive issues (such as constipation or gas), and sleep disturbance. Recovering mothers require support and receive these treatments:

- A daily massage with warm sesame oil is followed by a one-hour nap and a warm bath with leaves of tamarind, jackfruit, castor, and neem. All these have antimicrobial and antiviral properties. For the first week postbirth, a special treatment given after the normal massage is an herbal-leaf poultice massage, containing the leaves of the castor plant, tamarind, *Vitex negundo*, lime, and rock salt, which helps reduce body aches and improves muscle tone.
- Chyavanaprasham jam, shatavari, and ashwagandha are given as herbal tonics to restore the mother's energy and immunity and to promote high-quality breast milk.
- The diet is simple and bland, mainly vegetarian, consisting of light, warm soups and easily digestible foods, freshly and thoroughly cooked, especially for the first two weeks postpartum, with the heaviest meal at midday. Ghee (clarified butter) is used frequently.
- Large quantities of warm liquids, including purified water and boiled warm milk, are taken throughout the day and separately from meals to help rehydrate and warm the body.
- Much is done to promote a peaceful lifestyle and reduce stimulation with home-based rest—at least one month is considered ideal. This includes restricting the number of visitors and remaining in a warm, quiet environment sheltered from the cold and wind. Having others do domestic chores, including shopping, laundry, cooking, and cleaning, for at least a month is considered normal. Meditative and reflective activities such as yoga nidra are practiced twice daily. Exercise is minimal. Bedtime is early, usually by 9 p.m.

RESTORATIVE YOGA

There are many different forms of yoga, and they all have benefits, including improving mood; strengthening muscles and providing flexibility; encouraging mindfulness; and assisting and improving the function of the nervous system, immune system, and hormonal regulation. Although it is not considered one of the more traditional yogic practices, doing restorative yoga is an excellent way to regain your energy.

Restorative yoga involves the very gentle practice of placing your body in strategically supported positions, aided by bolsters, blankets, and other props. Combined with breathing exercises and the setting of intentions, this practice induces a restorative effect on your organs, circulation, immune system, and nearly every part of your body. Restorative yoga helps balance your autonomic nervous system (your body processes that are automatic, like your heart beating and your breathing) and encourages a rest-and-digest response to be activated. Scientists, in fact, have researched the effects of regular relaxation and report measurable benefits, including reduction in muscle tension and improved circulation. I suspect restorative yoga has important effects on helping to restore hormonal balance as well.

I learned about this amazing yoga style from the teachings of Judith Lasater, who is considered the queen of restorative yoga. In her many books, she has written poignantly about her own struggles with the challenges of motherhood and how important it was for her to have a letting-go—a literal grieving for her old life—which is essential for all mothers if they are to heal from their depletion and move forward with confidence and fulfillment in their new role as mothers.

A restorative yoga session is very gentle. You'll work on your breathing, and none of the poses are difficult for beginners. I suggest you take a few classes to master the basics, or even watch some of the many videos for free on YouTube, and then you will be able to do this wonderful form of yoga at home whenever you need to. It's an extremely effective way to reduce your tension and stress.

HOW TO DO LEGS UP THE WALL

According to Dr. Lauren Tober, a clinical psychologist and certified iRest yoga nidra teacher, the Viparita Karani (or Legs up the Wall Pose) is considered to be the ultimate restorative yoga posture. She suggests various yoga props, as well as alternatives you're likely to have around the house, but you can do this practice with no props at all if you need to.

- Start by placing a yoga mat (or blanket) on the floor, extending it out perpendicular from the wall. Place a bolster (or folded blanket) along the wall, leaving a small gap between the wall and the bolster. Experiment with different gaps to find the one that works best for you.
- Sit sideways on one end of your bolster, with one side of your body against the wall. Then gently lift both your legs up the wall, swiveling both hips evenly onto the bolster and resting your shoulders and head on the floor, so your legs are straight up the wall, and your body is perpendicular to the wall. This is usually a little awkward the first few times you do it, but it gets easier with practice!
- If your backside is away from the wall, lift your hips and use your shoulders to shuffle as close to the wall as possible, bringing your

How Restorative Yoga Works

The props (such as soft eye pillows, firm bolsters or pillows, a sturdy chair, and a wooden back bender for you to lie on) provide a totally supportive environment during your yoga session. They are an essential component of restorative yoga, as they help relieve your muscles and bones of their typical roles of support and/or action; this allows your body's nervous system to slow down and become calmer. It also lets you figure out where you hold on to the most tension in your body and allows you to concentrate on your breathing, which will permit you to become centered and present in the moment.

When you practice this form of yoga, you will be very slowly and gently backside to rest gently against or near the wall. With practice, you'll find the position that best suits your body.

- If it feels right, take a strap (or a scarf) and fasten it around your thighs, just below your knees, to hold your legs together. This will give you more support and increase your capacity to relax.
- Place an eye pillow (or a clean sock) over your eyes to gently rest your eyes and take your focus inward.
- Rest your palms on your abdomen and gently focus your attention on the rise and fall of your breath.
- Stay here for as long as feels comfortable, up to fifteen minutes. You might like to set a timer so you can deeply relax and not worry about the time.
- Make your way out of this posture very gently and slowly, by bringing your knees to your chest and slowly rolling off the bolster.
- If you have lower back pain or are menstruating, you might choose to do this posture without a bolster. Teachers are divided as to whether restorative Viparita Karani is good to practice while menstruating, so tune in to your body and decide if it feels good for you.

moving your spine in all directions, which will strengthen the muscles in your core. Doing inverted poses, such as Child's Pose and Legs up the Wall Pose, is good for your heart function and circulation. The poses alternately stimulate and soothe your internal organs, helping balance your energy.

BREATH AWARENESS, MEDITATION, AND BIOFEEDBACK

Learning how to relax is a skill like any other, and I hope that if you think about it this way, you'll be eager to learn what to do so you can wind yourself down when you need to. Paradoxically, the more relaxed you can become, the more this will restore your natural energy. This is because being in a relaxed state improves your circulation, especially by concentrating your blood flow toward your abdomen so your digestive and reproductive organs are nourished. And it also relieves so much of the stress that siphons off your energy just when you need it most.

Harvard-trained cardiologist and professor Herbert Benson coined the term "relaxation response" after discovering that you can calm yourself when you consciously let go of all thoughts and actively engage in a repetitive activity. A state of relaxation is when your nervous system is reset to a neutral position. There is no anticipation of stress, there is minimal physical tension, and levels of anxiety and worry are reduced.

Putting yourself into a state of relaxation is exactly what you do when you focus on your breathing and when you meditate. You use specific and easy-to-follow techniques in which you concentrate on each inhale and exhale, and this intense focus on such a simple yet profound act relaxes your entire body and helps your brain slow down and calm down.

Stress and the energy it zaps as a result are unavoidable; they're a part of life. In a lot of ways we need stress to get us up in the morning and motivated to do our jobs and raise our families—you already know that your cortisol level is at its highest in the morning when you've got to get your day sorted out. What's crucial is your response not just to normal everyday stress but also to the extraordinary and intense stress you have thanks to your postnatal depletion. You absolutely need to be able to switch off the stress and get to the relaxed state your body desperately needs.

This is particularly important because in your crazy-busy world of motherhood and postnatal depletion, relaxation time itself can actually be very stressful. Time alone can soon be filled with worries about the never-ending list of tasks you have to do, bills you have to pay, babysitters you have to find, baby-puke-covered clothing you have to wash, diapers you have to buy, food you have to cook, partner you have to talk to, colleagues and previous life you're trying to keep up with, and mother you catch giving you the stink-eye when she thinks you're not looking! Add baby brain into the mix and it's no wonder that you not only *can't* relax but don't *want* to relax either.

This is where conscious breathing, meditation, and biofeedback can be lifesavers. Once you learn how to relax properly and can click into relaxation mode whenever you need to (which is every day!), your relationship with stress will radically change. You will quickly be able to manage your stress and go from a meltdown to a well-balanced healthy juggling act.

How to Focus on Your Breathing

Focusing on your breathing helps bring about a sense of calm, and it reduces both physical and mental tension. Proper breathing is a simple yet powerful aid in stress reduction, detoxification, mindfulness, and

---

THE CORRECT WAY TO BREATHE

To become aware of your breathing pattern, place one hand on your chest and one hand on your abdomen. This can be done either seated or lying down. Then answer the following questions:

- Does your breath feel smooth or labored?
- Do you breathe through your nose or your mouth?
- Which hand moved first and most?
- Do your shoulders move as you breathe?
- Where is the tension or restriction in your breathing (jaw, face, belly, etc.)?
- Which is easier, your inhale or your exhale?
- Is the inhale full or does it stop somewhere in your body?

To see a natural breathing pattern, just watch your child breathe. You will see the belly naturally rise and fall. We see this because the diaphragm is the primary breathing muscle and it is pulling the air deep down into the body, expanding the tummy, ribs, and lower back. The pattern should be two-thirds diaphragmatic, and the final third should be chest movement:

As you inhale, your belly should rise.

At the same time, you should feel your lower ribs and back expand, almost like a round cylinder. Ideally, your shoulders remain relaxed.

The last place to move is your upper chest.

---

bodily awareness. It also helps maintain the acid/alkaline (or pH) balance of your body, removes waste, and supports a more restful sleep at night. It also resets your system to get you back on track.

We breathe around 20,000 times per day, yet most of us are not aware of the mechanics. Rushing around or feeling stressed causes the breath to become more shallow. Highly stressed people are often "chest breathers" who don't breathe deeply into the belly. Chest breathing is problematic because it makes the muscles around the neck and upper chest excessively tight, as they are forced to perform a task they are not made for.

If you are chronically unable to breathe through your nose, you may want to investigate allergies or food intolerances, such as to dairy or gluten. These can cause inflammation, and your body's response to

THE FOUR-IN/SEVEN-OUT BREATHING TECHNIQUE

Here's my favorite breathing exercise, which I learned from a well-known cardiologist in San Diego, Dr. Mimi Guarneri. She teaches it to her highly stressed cardiac patients as a relaxation technique. The best part about it is that you can do it anywhere, anytime, whether you're driving your car, standing in an interminably long line at the supermarket, or rocking your baby to sleep. Practicing this simple technique for thirty to sixty seconds can make a huge difference in your current stress state.

All you do is breathe in through your nose to a count of four, and breathe out through your nose to a count of seven. Breathe evenly without force. The evenness on the out breath is what will calm you down and relax you the most, so you need to focus on stretching out the exhale so that not all the air comes out in the first part of the counting. With very little practice, you'll exhale perfectly to the count of seven and will reap the benefits in no time.

that may include the formation of excess mucus that blocks your nasal passages.

Remember, as you become more repleted and start getting back into movement and regular exercise, your breath is always there, readily available, to help you move your *qi* throughout all parts of your body. It's a simple but powerful tool that is always there for you!

HELP WITH SHALLOW BREATHING

If your breathing feels labored or shallow, here is an exercise that will make it easier. Remember that it will take some practice to ingrain this new habit.

- Lie down with one hand on your chest and one hand on your belly. Keep your knees bent, or stretch out your legs and position a pillow beneath your knees.
- As you inhale through your nose, see if you can make your tummy rise by using your diaphragm, while keeping the shoulders and neck as relaxed as possible.
- Once you have the hang of this, see if you can feel your lower ribs move sideways as you inhale. You can feel for this by placing your hands on your lower ribs.
- Finally, visualize your breath coming all the way into your abdomen, lower ribs, *and lower back*, almost like a round cylinder. Ideally, the shoulders and neck should remain relaxed throughout. The movement is one of allowing rather than forcing.

Once you have this pattern down, with your belly rising on the inhale before the chest rises, you can try the following: See if you can feel the support of the floor, mat, or bed underneath you. If so, can you allow yourself to rest into it and feel the support underneath you? Ask yourself if you are holding yourself up somewhere or feeling tension. Then allow yourself to soften into those areas, using your breath to let go of any tension, physical or emotional. What does that feel like? Hopefully, it feels wonderful!

How to Meditate

Meditation is a truly wonderful thing to do for yourself. All you need is a quiet room and a few minutes—you will reap the benefits even if you can spare only a minute or two. Basically you sit in a comfortable position and focus on your breathing. When you are relaxed, you can either follow a creative visualization—picturing something in your mind's eye, such as an intense beam of light or focusing on something you would like to create in your life, such as strength or wellness—or repeat a mantra that will give your brain a chance to relax. You can find guided meditations online or download apps to your phone that will walk you through different meditative exercises for whatever your intentions or needs, and they will always make you feel better.

Meditation rules change once you become a mother, however, and you find both time and quiet rooms to be in short supply! Even if your baby could talk, I don't think you'd hear him suggest, "Hey, Mommy, why don't you take five minutes to do an undisturbed, relaxing meditation?" So you'll need to be a little creative about carving out some time and space for yourself. When I'm very busy, I often find myself doing breathing techniques while waiting in traffic or standing in line at the supermarket. If I can steal away, I'll take two to five minutes, sitting in a chair or lying on the ground, and do the meditation on the next page. It can be done with or without your baby. If you find you are too tired and keep nodding off, then you should take a micronap instead.

How to Use Biofeedback

Biofeedback uses devices to measure your internal signals, such as heart rate, and displays these signals externally on a computer screen or smartphone. This can be fascinating and incredibly valuable feedback, especially for mothers who are juggling multiple responsibilities at all times. You might be feeling okay, for example, but if you see that your body is actually in the middle of a stress response, you can take steps to change what you're doing.

MY FAVORITE MEDITATION

Sit comfortably or lie down, close your eyes, and gently get in touch with your body. Notice any physical tension or discomfort. Also notice any feelings of sadness or vulnerability. Accept that these feelings are present; accept, too, as with all things, that they will pass.

Breathe in deeply and slowly, and then breathe out deeply and slowly.

Breathing in and out through your nose to a count of four is a useful start. If you want to elongate the breathing pattern, while you're counting silently to yourself, space out your count of four by adding the number ninety-nine in between each of the four counts. Breathe in "one ninety-nine two ninety-nine three ninety-nine four ninety-nine." Then breathe out "one ninety-nine two ninety-nine three ninety-nine four ninety-nine."

With each in breath, imagine a color from a sunrise—pink, red, or orange (this can change with each breath). With each out breath, imagine the sun's rays touching your body and surrounding you with their golden light. (The colors on the in breath can change as the sun rises, but the color that enters your body is always golden light.)

With each in breath, feel the relaxation and calm enter your body. With each out breath, feel the anxiety, overwhelm, and worry leave your body.

As you finish, open your eyes and take a few more slow breaths. With each in breath, think, "Life is good." With each out breath, think, "I feel at peace."

As you finish, take a moment to feel gratitude for all the love and caring that surrounds you on your amazing journey as a mom.

One way to relax is through "cardiac coherence training," which is particularly useful if you have anxiety or are in energy-zapping stress overload. The way you do this is with a biofeedback device or app that measures the moment-to-moment changes in your heart rate variability (HRV) so you can see just how your body is reacting to your environment. I encourage moms to check their HRV when they're waiting for something, such as your child at school pickup, sports training, or dance class. Once you've loaded a biofeedback app or program on any of your electronic devices, you can check your HRV and use this information to get yourself back into a positive relaxation state.

Using a Biofeedback/HRV Device or App

The easiest and most portable biofeedback option I recommend is HeartMath, an amazing device that syncs with the Inner Balance Trainer app for your smartphone. A sensor that fits over your finger or on your ear measures your HRV and then, if needed, you are guided through either breathing techniques or visualizations that will help you get into a more relaxed and emotionally coherent state. The app provides suggestions and coaching, and you can use it for as long or as short a time as you like. Many mothers find it beneficial to use this app for five minutes twice per day or when they are dealing with something very stressful.

CHLOE'S REGIMEN

Chloe was a twenty-nine-year-old mother of an eighteen-month-old toddler and was eight weeks pregnant with her second child. She'd had a "dreadful" first pregnancy, with poor energy and depression, and she wanted to be happier and feel better with this new pregnancy.

What the Testing Showed

Chloe was anemic, with low iron and blood protein, skewed copper and zinc levels, low homocysteine, and low DHEA.

Chloe's Protocol

Due to Chloe's pregnancy, I was limited in what supplements and interventions would be safe for her to use. She was already on a good prenatal supplement, and I added DHA, zinc, pyrrole correction, NAC, bone broths, and protein powder. The psychologist whom Chloe went to see was trained in iRest yoga nidra, and part of Chloe's treatment included several prerecorded meditation exercises to do for thirty minutes every other day.

Chloe reported that initially she found it very challenging to find the time to do this, but once she got into the habit she was able to do it every day, and she soon greatly looked forward to "her time" with this technique. In her second trimester, she started on ashwagandha as an adaptogenic herb. By twenty weeks, she was feeling great and had a very positive experience with her pregnancy and beyond.

CHAPTER 8

Rebuilding Sleep

When was the last time you woke up from a blissful, deep, completely refreshing full night's sleep?

If you're like most of my patients, getting enough sleep is as tangible as a distant memory. In fact, as you know already, lack of sleep has a terrible effect on your vibrancy, health, and well-being. You can't digest your food properly and you can't hit the reset button on your energy. Your production of cortisol, the stress hormone, is out of whack. This is not a situation that can be ignored, because the less you sleep, the worse you feel about everything going on in your life.

If you still have a child waking up during the night, it will be hard to truly recuperate from sleep deprivation. Believe me, I know how difficult this period can be, and there is literature out there about how to help transition your child into sleeping through the night. But while I cannot sit through the night with your child so that you can get your much-needed rest, I can give you some advice on how to make the sleep that you are getting more impactful.

In chapter 2, you learned that many physical changes take place in your brain when you're pregnant. While these changes prepare you to bond with and care for your infant by making you hypervigilant, the downside is the hijacking of sleep quality. Combined with seemingly endless nighttime feeding rituals, havoc is wreaked on your much-needed sleep cycle. Deep sleep is nature's built-in stress-reduction mechanism. The brain cycles through various sleep stages over a ninety-minute period, progressing into deeper and deeper states of sleep. Disturb the cycle and the little sleep you manage to get will not be restorative but instead will leave you feeling like a zombie.

If you want to drive someone crazy, a surefire way to do so is by continually waking them up, especially during periods of deep sleep. Just ask those who torture or interrogate in prisons—it's a time-tested tactic that makes the innocent confess to crimes they never committed just so they can go back to sleep.

Ideally, when you start yawning in the evening, you want to brush your teeth and sink into a lovely, comfortable bed, safe in the knowledge that you're going to sleep well. When you're depleted and exhausted, however, you experience a big change in the architecture of your sleep. If you're so tired that you nod off when don't expect to—in a classroom, while watching TV, even while breastfeeding the baby—you're not getting rejuvenating deep sleep, and whatever shuteye you did manage to achieve, you'll still feel as if you hadn't slept at all!

HOW TO GET THE RESTFUL SLEEP YOU NEED

I've devised a system so you can finally get the deep, restorative sleep you need. These recommendations are based both on my clinical observation and on the rapidly growing body of sleep science. Try to follow as many of these tips as you can. As a starting point, I advise my patients to go through the list and choose to work on suggestions that are most easily achievable. Your sleep should start to improve within a few nights, with progressive benefits over the following weeks. Good sleep begets good sleep. I promise that even as you are dealing with being up with your child one (or more) times a night, these changes will improve the quality of the sleep that you are able to get.

1. *Limit Exposure to Blue Light an Hour before You Go to Sleep*

What does blue light have to do with achieving deep sleep? Well, it all has to do with your pineal gland—which has a lot to answer for when it comes to your sleep!

The pineal gland is a tiny organ found in the middle of your brain. Its primary function is to release melatonin, the hormone that is responsible for regulating your circadian rhythm—your unique internal body clock, which determines your sleep/wake cycle over a twenty-four-hour period. It also helps regulate some of your reproductive hormones, but what's important now is for you to think of melatonin as the sleep hormone.

Where do the pineal gland's instructions come from? The answer is that we just don't know for certain. We *do* know that melatonin's release is triggered by exposure to light, in the form of sunshine and internal lighting. Before electricity was discovered, most people's sleep cycles were determined by nature; melatonin levels were low during the day and increased as soon as it got dark. But in modern life we spend far less time in natural light and far more time in artificial light than the human body was ever used to before.

So what does this have to do with blue light and you not sleeping? Well, scientists have recently discovered that the pineal gland, which receives its information directly from the eye, is very sensitive to the 472 nm spectrum of blue light. In prehistoric times, blue light came only from the sun, and the closer to midday it was, the bluer the light. This wavelength tells the pineal gland that it's daytime; your body interprets this information as a signal to release cortisol for energy, not melatonin for sleep.

Now, of course, blue light comes from many sources: lightbulbs (including many but not all energy-saving lightbulbs), computer screens, mobile devices, and TV sets. You're staring at blue light all day long—and well into the night, too. This tricks your body out of its true day/night cycle and disrupts your circadian rhythm.

What to Do:

- Wear orange-tinted glasses with a blue-light filter for 1 hour before "bedtime." These were initially designed for use at a computer, they're inexpensive, and they can easily be found online. They might not be the most fashionable eyewear you've ever owned, but they work!

- Install software on your computer that will orange-tint your screen as the evening progresses. It remains as blue light during the day and gradually shifts as nighttime approaches. One company that offers this download (free for those using Macs/Linux/Windows) is F.lux. Another is called Iris.
- Install night-friendly lightbulbs with a yellow or orange hue in your bedroom, at the very least, but also in the rooms where you spend a lot of time before going to sleep. This will be good not just for you but for all your family members as well. A salt lamp will provide the right spectrum of light to assist sleep.
- Ensure that your room is as dark as possible. Install blackout curtains on the windows. If you need to leave a night-light on to help guide you when you get up for nighttime feedings, use a soft sleep mask made from cotton, silk, or bamboo fibers.
- In the morning, you want to expose your body to full-spectrum or natural sunlight for fifteen minutes between 8 a.m. and 10 a.m. without sunglasses or glasses on. Outside is ideal; if you're inside, open as many windows as possible because you can't get this full spectrum of light through glass. You need to get this light to your pineal gland, which, as you know, is done via your eyes. You shouldn't need to wear sunscreen during this very short period unless you are very prone to sunburn.

2. *Improve Your Sleep Hygiene*

Sleep hygiene has nothing to do with being clean or dirty! It's a medical concept used to describe your typical routine in the hour before going to bed. Think of this as a global dimming switch for your senses. The hour before sleep is critical in regulating your circadian rhythm; use this time to help induce and maintain sleep.

Scientists and sleep researchers often toss around phrases like "reducing the intensity of one's environment," but what they really mean is that you need to deliberately wind down. Try to set up a bedtime ritual. It will be easy to follow after a while and will tell your brain that you're serious about going to bed! In addition to getting rid of the blue light on any of your electronics, consider the following tips.

What to Do:

- Reduce noise in the home. If you live in a noisy area, consider a white-noise machine or just a plain old box fan, which can help block out irregular or annoying noise from outside.
- Avoid physical activity that elevates your heart rate for an extended period for at least two hours before bed. The good news is that intimacy and sex are not considered exercise; they are, in fact, beneficial for sleep (but more on that in chapter 13).
- Try to avoid emotionally stimulating activities prior to sleep. This includes social media, intense movies or TV shows, and news programs. One silly or enraging posting on Facebook is enough to wake up your tired brain and prevent you from getting the good-quality sleep you crave. This also means you should try to have any important discussions with your partner long before bedtime, because you don't want any talks to spill into your needed sleep time. Try not to have a TV in the bedroom, and turn off your computer, tablets, and phone.
- Read a good book—not an upsetting book like the history of serial killers, of course, but a book that gives you pleasure. Many of my patients tell me that they get through only a few pages before they conk out and that it takes them months to finish their book, but that makes me happy—it means that they're falling right asleep!
- Take a soak in a hot bath or even a foot bath. The warmth is a great way to help your body relax. You can increase this effect by adding magnesium sulfate bath salts to the water.
- The ideal temperature for sleep is between 60 and 68 degrees Fahrenheit. This is a lot cooler than you might be used to, especially in homes with central heating. If you're used to sleeping in a hot room, gradually turn down the thermostat a

degree or two until you adjust to the change. It's much better to sleep in a cool room with a lot of blankets than in a warmer room with one blanket. Our core temperature during our deepest sleep drops 3 to 4 degrees Fahrenheit below baseline, so if your room is too hot, it's harder for your body to reduce its core temperature to achieve this deep sleep state, as anyone who has slept in a hot room can testify.

- Your bedroom should be a haven of comfort for you. Try to keep it as uncluttered as possible. Keep your closet doors closed. Have a decent air flow; you never want your bedroom to feel stuffy. A good mattress is a must to properly support your body. Use the best-quality bedding you can afford, made out of natural fibers, which will help your body stay at a normal temperature (synthetic fibers can cause you to sweat during the night). Find pillows that are the right softness/hardness you like—everyone's taste is different. I also advise either using allergy pillow protectors or changing your pillow every eighteen months due to the accumulation of dust mites that can occur in nonlatex pillows.

3. *Try Alternative and Meditative Therapies*

I am a huge proponent of holistic and alternative methods for relaxation and better sleep. There is no downside to doing any of these techniques. They'll improve not only your sleep but your overall health as well.

What to Do:

Acupuncture. Not only does acupuncture help with postnatal depletion, as you learned already, but it can be used specifically for insomnia and sleep problems.

Meditation. Meditation, as you learned in chapter 7, is a wonderful way to calm your thought processes and regulate your breathing, so it can be incredibly helpful in pushing you past those thoughts and stresses that cause you to toss and turn at night.

HOW TO DO YOGA NIDRA

This sequence is shared by yoga teacher Dr. Lauren Tober.

- Lie down in any comfortable position, and place a cushion under your head. If you're lying on your back, place a yoga bolster or a rolled-up blanket under your knees. Cover your body with a blanket, and place an eye pillow or clean sock over your eyes.
- Gently state your intention for the practice, affirming it in the positive and present tense, such as *I am deeply relaxed* or *I welcome whatever arises.*
- Spend a few moments opening to each of your senses. Notice sounds. Smells. Taste. Color or light behind your eyelids. The touch of the air on your skin.
- Rotate your attention around your body, feeling and noticing whatever sensations are present, without expectation or judgment. Feel your body from the inside rather than looking with your eyes. If there are no sensations, simply feel what the absence of sensation feels like.
- Start by noticing sensation in your mouth. Then notice sensation in your left ear, right ear, and both ears at the same time. Do the same with your eyes.

Yoga Nidra. Yoga nidra is not the same as restorative yoga. Instead, it's a deeply restorative mindfulness meditation that is invaluable to depleted and exhausted moms. It's done while you're lying down, and your instructor will guide you into a state of deep relaxation—the brain-wave state closest to the sleep state. Regular sessions can teach you how to drift off into slumber; reduce depression, stress, and worries; lessen chronic and acute pain; and increase your feelings of inner peace, relaxation, and well-being.

Stretching. Gentle stretching before bed for ten to fifteen minutes has been shown to be beneficial in relaxing your body in preparation for

- Notice sensation in your forehead, scalp, back of the head, neck, and throat.
- Notice sensation in your left arm, starting at the shoulder and moving down to the hand, then the whole left arm. Do the same with your right arm; then sense both arms at the same time.
- Sense the front of the torso, the back of the torso, and then the entire torso.
- Notice sensation in the left leg, starting at the hip and moving down to the toes, and then the whole left leg. Do the same with the right leg; then sense both legs at the same time.
- Sense the entire body, inside and out.
- Notice the rise and fall of your abdomen as you breathe. Try counting your breaths, slowly and rhythmically backward from nine to one.
- Rest in comfort and relaxation for as long as you like. Before you finish up, spend a few moments imagining yourself going about your daily life, bringing this quality of relaxation and ease to every moment of your day.
- State your intention again to yourself and notice if another intention arises for your next practice or for the rest of your day.
- Express gratitude to yourself, for taking the time to practice yoga nidra.

sleep and in helping you stay asleep. Ask a certified physical therapist or physical trainer to give you a pre-bedtime routine.

Aromatherapy. Aromatherapy is the use of essential oils extracted from plants and flowers, each with a specific therapeutic purpose. It has been used across cultures for centuries as a way of helping relax the recovering mother and to improve her sleep. Essential oils are highly concentrated and can be used several different ways.

- To use in a full-body bath, add up to 5 drops essential oil to a tub of warm water. For a foot bath, add 2 to 3 drops to the warm water.

- For a massage, use a 2.5 percent dilution of the essential oil to your carrier oil, such as sweet almond, jojoba, or argan oil. This is about 5 drops essential oil for every 2 teaspoons carrier oil.
- For inhalation, the best way to use essential oils is by diffusing them. Diffusers are easy to find online, and you need to add only a few drops to the water each time you use a diffuser.

Because essential oils are so concentrated, they should never be used directly on skin, and a little goes a very long way. Have fun with them, and get creative making customized blends. A personalized formula would be a great gift to give other recovering mothers.

THE BEST AROMATHERAPY OILS FOR SLEEP

- Lavender is used for its calming effect.
- Bergamot, sweet orange, and tangerine oils have a positive effect in improving sleep quality in the postpartum period.
- Fragonia, part of the eucalyptus family, is a unique Australian essential oil that induces a profound feeling of calmness and tranquility and a genuine feeling of serenity. It blends well with oils such as lavender, clary sage, neroli, and sandalwood to offer a lifting and calming effect.
- Patchouli, ylang ylang, and rose geranium are used for calming and balancing.

4. *Change Your Before-Bedtime Eating and Drinking Habits*

What to Do:

- Try not to eat a large meal for at least two hours before bedtime. While you might sometimes like a nap after a large lunch, a nighttime meal will definitely affect your sleeping. Your body uses the sleeping hours to do the grunt work of digestion, but if you have a lot of food in your stomach, especially carbohydrates that affect your blood sugar levels, your body will need to use a lot of energy just to digest and manage that food, and this can keep you up or wake you up.

- If you are hungry before bed, the best thing to eat is a small protein-based snack. Insulin, which regulates your blood sugar, is not released in response to protein-only foods. Fluctuating blood sugar can evoke the "stress" response in many people, causing them to wake more easily and have a harder time getting back to sleep.
- Try taking caprylic acid (medium-chain triglyceride, or MCT, oil from coconuts). This has a stabilizing effect on your blood sugar, which greatly improves calmness in your brain while you're sleeping. Start with 1 teaspoon initially and slowly increase to the full dose of 1 tablespoon.
- Drink caffeinated beverages only in the morning, not after midday. Check the caffeine levels in your decaf drinks, too—you might be unpleasantly surprised to find out that certain teas or decaf brands of coffee have a lot more caffeine in them than you realized!
- A hot drink without calories like an herbal tea is ideal before bedtime. Herbs such as chamomile, valerian, lavender, lemon balm, peppermint, and St. John's wort are all well-known relaxants and sleep inducers. At our clinic, we also recommend chamomile tea for babies over the age of two months. To make it, steep the chamomile for five minutes, cool it to body temperature or slightly cooler, and then put 1 to 2 ounces in a baby bottle. Give it once a day, and once it's well tolerated it can be used more often.
- Avoid alcohol for at least two hours before bed. While you may think that a drink will help you relax and fall asleep more quickly, in certain parts of the brain, it can act as a stimulant and can disrupt deep sleep; the higher the level of alcohol in your system, the more

it can affect your quality of sleep—not what mothers in a delicate state of postnatal recovery need.

- Try not to drink too much water before bedtime so you don't wake up to pee. If you do need to use the bathroom, use an incandescent lightbulb or a night-light that gives off a soft yellow, orange, or even red hue to keep your pineal gland from mistaking night for day!

5. *Try Supplements once Your Health-Care Practitioner Gives You the Okay*

Supplements can be useful when used correctly and when needed. Obviously, you don't need to take all of these at the same time. Just as obviously, you should never self-diagnose what and how much to take of any supplements. My advice is to find a holistic practitioner, such as a naturopathic or functional doctor and/or licensed herbalist, who can help you, especially to ensure that your breast milk won't be adversely affected, and always tell your obstetrician and/or gynecologist what you are taking. Some mainstream doctors are hostile or not well informed about these supplements, but I have been prescribing them for my patients for more than ten years, and I know they can help tremendously with sleep.

What to Do:

If you are feeling tense, if your mind won't stop racing or fretting, or if you are having trouble winding down or getting into a relaxed state before bedtime, consider nutraceuticals:

- Seeking Health's optimal liposomal magnesium, 10 ml 30 minutes before bed. This is great for relaxing muscles and then in turn relaxing the mind.
- Quicksilver's liposomal GABA with L-theanine, 4 sprays before bed. This is good for reducing racing thoughts and calming the brain.
- Melatonin, 1 mg 30 minutes before bed. This can be immensely useful for insomnia, but talk to a qualified health practitioner before taking it.

If your adrenal glands need assistance, consider taking adrenal-boosting herbs:

- Organic India's ashwagandha, 800 mg twice a day. Taking this during the day has been shown to help with the ability to get to sleep at night. I particularly like this herb because it is well tolerated and effective and has a very long cultural use going back thousands of years within traditional Indian culture.
- 5-HTP, any brand, 50 to 100 mg before bed. This is the precursor amino acid to serotonin and melatonin. Do *not* take this if you are on any antidepressants.

Herbal remedies for sleeping have been used for generations, but surprisingly little research has been done on their safety for pregnant and lactating mothers. My preferred combination product in terms of both effect and safety with long-term use includes valerian (300 mg), passionflower (80 mg), and hops (30 mg). If this isn't working, then I typically use a slightly higher dose, such as that found in Flordis's ReDormin. Or try these:

- Valerian, 0.75 to 1.25 g per dose, 30 minutes before bed. Valerian has been shown to help reduce anxiety and help promote a feeling of tiredness and calm. Hops, 360 mg per oral dose, 30 minutes before bed. Hops have a long history and can be used in various ways: a hops bath with a few drops of concentrated extract added to the bathwater, an oral dosage, or a hops-infused tea.
- Passionflower and skullcap are often used in sleep formulas for mothers, as is chamomile (although chamomile is more for relaxation than for inducing sleep).
- Ashwagandha, 800 mg twice a day. This adrenal herb, mentioned previously, is one of my frontline herbs for fatigue, and it also helps the body tolerate the negative consequences of sleep deprivation.

6. *Make Decisions about Breastfeeding*

Whether or not you are cosleeping with your baby, it is important to know how much broken sleep you're getting. One important aspect that many of my mothers don't want to discuss but need to, especially if they are severely depleted, is when to end breastfeeding. This is a loaded topic—entire books have been written about it!

The World Health Organization (WHO) recommends breastfeeding until the age of two, but for a mom with postnatal depletion, six to twelve months is sufficient. If you need to stop breastfeeding because you're depleted (or for any other reason), especially if the baby is older than one year, then *you should stop*!

I know how difficult this topic is. Breastfeeding can be one of the most wonderful and intimate bonding experiences a mother and baby can have, and ending it can be emotionally wrenching. I make a point about not telling my patients how to parent but to assist them in their parental decision-making. I think it's important for mothers to make the connection between nursing and their own sleep deprivation. How I frame this issue in my clinic is specifically around improving sleep for the mother, not any other factors. I will either support them through this or send them to a lactation/sleep consultant, especially if the baby is under nine months of age.

All too often, mothers who come to see me in a state of terrible depletion admit that their babies are older than twelve months yet are still nursing at night, sometimes for nutrition and sometimes for comfort suckling, not for a sizable meal. Often the baby may not even fully awaken from his or her slumber and is practically on autopilot searching for the comforting nipple—and this, of course, wakes Mommy from her precious deep slumber. There is nothing inherently wrong with comfort suckling, but if you feel frazzled and exhausted, this in the long term does not serve anyone, including the baby. There are other ways that babies can learn to comfort themselves.

What to Do:

- If you're having trouble with this issue, speak to your doctor or a health-care professional who can advise you. It may seem daunting to change your routine, even though you know the nighttime awakenings are furthering your depletion, but the right professional guidance can help.
- You should also be aware that whenever breastfeeding ends, there are hormonal changes that can make you feel emotionally low for several days until your body adjusts. This is very normal and passes quickly. If you expect these changes, they can be much easier to manage. I recommend keeping nonessential activities and socializing to a minimum when you do end breastfeeding so that you can give yourself the space you need.

7. *Reduce Electromagnetic Fields in Your Environment*

Studies about the effects of electro-smog are being reported in scientific literature as well as by the media. Electro-smog refers to the combined additive effects of all the electrical and magnetic fields in our modern environment. Not only does this include mobile phones, wireless internet, and electrical appliances; it also takes into account the quality of the electricity itself that's being delivered to our homes and the quality of the wiring inside our homes, which produce potentially the most harmful of all the electromagnetic-field (EMF) signals: dirty electricity.

EMFs can be hard to understand, especially as they're invisible. I prefer the term *electro-smog*, as it brings to mind images of air pollution. If you live in an isolated country house, your air is likely to be clean and free from smog; if you live in a crowded city, your air is likely to be severely polluted. Same with electro-smog. If you are living in the countryside far from other houses, you will likely have fewer issues with EMFs than you would if you lived in a densely populated urban area, where you are exposed not only to your own EMFs but also to those of the many people around you.

Evidence is mounting that EMFs contribute to inflammation by causing an influx of calcium into the cells. This intracellular calcium, which shouldn't be there, requires energy to remove and causes inflammation in the process. Because EMFs are presumed to be safe by regulators, the public assumes they are safe. Yet with increasing disease rates in every direction, it is practically impossible to know how much of a factor EMFs have on human bodies. After discussing this with my patients for years, I have come to believe that for those who are particularly susceptible—and certainly for those with postnatal depletion—sleep can be affected by EMFs in your home. Simple changes can make an enormous difference.

What to Do:

- Turn off your modem before you go to bed, and either turn off all your devices, including phones and tablets, or put them in airplane mode.
- Turn off and unplug anything that isn't essential for the overnight functioning of the house.
- As a test, shut off all the electricity for your house at the fuse box overnight to see if your sleep improves. I have a number of patients who've had their good-quality sleep magically returned to them by doing exactly this. (Keep a flashlight by the bed, and turn your refrigerator on as soon as you wake up; a few hours shouldn't affect what's in the fridge as long as you keep the doors closed. Just to be safe, take all the items in your freezer, especially any precious breast milk you may have, to a neighbor's freezer overnight, so you don't worry about it.) If you find that this really makes a difference, you can have an electrician install a separate switch at the main fuse box just for the fridge and freezer, so the whole house can get switched off at night, apart from the refrigeration.

8. *Get Earthing!*

I'm certain that the primary reason people feel good when they spend time at the beach is not the lovely view or the warming sun but the high density of electrons found there. On the surface of the water, especially where there is movement of water over the earth—such as in a river or with wave action at the ocean—the electron densities are greatly increased. Every process in our bodies needs electrons, and if we do not have enough of them, this affects our ability to deal with inflammation quickly and contributes in part to lethargy, disrupted sleep cycles, and our inability to concentrate and think clearly. "Earthing" is about giving your body access to electrons in a beneficial way—and our only source of electrons is being in physical contact with the earth's electrical field. Because our bodies are electrically charged, we will respond in a beneficial way to the natural electrons that are constantly flowing from the planet we live on.

As humans evolved, we were never *not* in contact with the earth's electrical field. We initially went barefoot but continued to spend a lot of time outside even as our footwear improved. In this modern age of wearing rubber-soled shoes, living in insulated homes, walking on concrete roads, and interacting constantly with electronic devices, we can go without contact with the earth's electrical field for days on end. As a result, I believe that we can suffer from an electron deficiency.

This is not an out-there crazy theory but a new and underfunded field of research. I have so many patients tell me they sleep better and have more energy when they start earthing. It is my belief that it's not so much that earthing can give them new energy but instead that their cells are now able to function better.

To do your own unofficial test for electron deficiency, go to the beach and keep your feet on damp sand or in shallow water for thirty minutes. This is how long it takes your body to get a full electron flush from head to foot. If you feel better, with more energy and regained vitality, alertness, and life, then earthing is for you.

What to Do:

- Walk barefoot or with leather soles on bare earth (or to a lesser extent concrete) as much as possible.
- Spend as much time at the beach (or lake or river—wherever a large body of water meets land) as possible. That's right: Doctor's orders are to take a beach day!

- Use an earthing sheet on your bed. For me, an earthing sheet is one of the easiest and least expensive investments you can make for your long-term health. It is simply a cotton fitted sheet with silver thread woven through it and is meant to be plugged in to an electrical socket.
- Use an earthing mat at your computer desk under your keyboard, or placed on the floor for your feet. It's the same technique as using an earthing sheet.

APRIL'S REGIMEN

I saw April, age thirty-five, when her older child was two and her baby was seven months old.

Her symptom list was long and she was really struggling. She felt like she was being woken up many times during the night and then had trouble getting back to sleep. Her husband was away a lot for work, both kids slept in the bed with her, and she felt she'd never recovered from either birth and was in a total fog. "I'm so tired and have no energy. My eyes are always burning, I'm light-headed, and I'm craving sweets all the time," she told me. "My batteries are flat. But I want a realistic plan. I tried supplements before and I had a hard time remembering to take them because I didn't feel like they were doing me any good."

What the Testing Showed

April had low vitamin B_{12}, high copper, and low DHEA.

April's Protocol

April's plan for six weeks included intravenous vitamin C, DHEA daily, a high dose of ashwagandha, and a single intramuscular dose of vitamin B_{12}. I convinced her to rearrange her bedroom so that there were three beds at the same level, which made breastfeeding easier at night (she could then transfer the baby to the crib). I also told her to switch off the

Wi-Fi at night and stop all social media use, get an earthing sheet for her bed, put a Himalayan salt lamp in her bedroom, and try lavender-based aromatherapy for her bedtime wind-down. I also convinced her to stick to the supplements, if only for a few weeks, and she was so exhausted she didn't protest!

Six weeks later, April was a different person, fully refreshed and happily telling me how helpful the supplements actually were. In addition, now that she was sleeping better through these interventions and had, as she put it, her "brain back," she had a lightbulb moment and realized how much support she needed. She met up with other mothers, got a cleaner, asked her mother-in-law and babysitters to take the kids more often, and engaged in activities that she wanted to do when her partner wasn't home—all remedies she'd never entertained before.

PART III

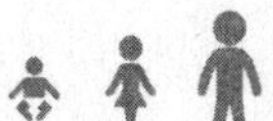

The Second and Third Trimesters: Completing Physical Recovery

CHAPTER 9

The Optimal Energy Food Plan

Now that you've learned how to treat your postnatal depletion with micronutrients and macronutrients, hormones, alternative treatments, and better sleep, let me show you how to eat. These are the food plans I give to my patients, and I know they work. I have worked closely with nutritionists and naturopaths for many years to develop these guidelines for my patients, and you can find more information on my website about shopping lists and meal planning.

As you read this chapter, I want you to think about the challenges you face when it comes to getting the right food into your house and into your body. Cooking is difficult when you are depleted and exhausted and much more so when you first have to go grocery shopping with the baby in tow.

In my practice, I discuss with my patients the basic guidelines that you'll read in this chapter, work out each of their individual needs, and then refer them to our nutritionist, who devises meal plans with them and helps create the shopping lists. (I've found that victushealth.com, as an example, is a useful website to aid in meal-planning.) There is simply no one-size-fits-all approach, as every woman has different levels of depletion, but it is possible for everyone to make good, nourishing food out of fast and easy ingredients. I give you a lot of hacks, too, that instantly boost the nutritional value of your diet. You should start feeling better in only a week, with long-lasting benefits after six weeks.

EATING THE SAPIEN WAY

In a world of junk food, we all need support in becoming smarter about our food. I use an acronym that is easy to remember for the way I want you to think about food: SAPIEN. *Sapien* is the Latin word for "wise" or "smart."

S Is for Supplement-Enhanced and Superfoods

You know that when you're depleted, you will likely need micronutrient supplements to help you recover. Once you're on the road to recovery, the *S* will refer to superfoods. These are foods that are particularly high in nutrients, making them almost supplement-like in nature. See the list on page 170 for suggestions.

A Is for Anthropologically Appropriate

There are certain foods and combinations of foods that are culturally based, and these may be dishes that you grew up eating and particularly like. This partly has to do with our genetic and ethnic makeups. But the foods we ate during childhood also played a major role in setting up our microbiomes, the bacterial populations that live within our large intestine. This is why Asians, for example, are less likely to tolerate a diet rich in dairy, while French, Italians, and Greeks do better with the Mediterranean style of eating (fresh veggies, limited protein, and olive oil). An important part of cultural eating centers on families coming together to share a meal and enjoy one another's company. It should be a time of connection. I have always tried to do this with my children—sharing food, sharing stories, checking in with one another. It is, however, vastly challenging trying to remain in a state of joy and connection when kids are being, well, kids; they often don't want to eat and leave the food on the plate or, worse, on the floor. Mealtimes can sometimes feel more like a circus performance than a coming together of a loving, respectful family unit.

P Is for Paleo Inspired

Paleolithic eating is a more traditional type of food preparation. This diet describes a way of eating that uses foods stemming from preagricultural times, when humans were principally hunter-gatherers. What is certain is that our Paleolithic ancestors did not eat grains, dairy, and legumes in any large amount, so a strict Paleo diet avoids those foods. I certainly am not so rigid about the consumption of dairy and legumes; while these foods can be inflammatory for many people, I do not see this as a black-and-white rule. I believe each person needs to discover which types of dairy and legumes might be okay for them and then be open to exploring a new diet that might better support what the depleted body needs.

I use Paleo ideas and recipes as an inspiring way to eat the simple foods that our ancestors were familiar with and to prepare them in a wholesome, simple way. The Paleo diet prohibits grains, favoring instead quality proteins and the liberal consumption of healthy fats.

I Is for Individualized

The idea of individualized diets respects that there is no one diet or one eating philosophy that is best for all people. Much of the diet advice out there, as you likely know, takes a generic one-size-fits-all approach and is based on population science. I find that a lot of people feel disempowered when it comes to scolding dietary advice. They may feel fine eating something they "shouldn't" (according to popular cultural thinking), or they may not feel well fueled eating something that is meant to be good for them. Individualizing your diet, especially with professional guidance and nutritional expertise, means identifying foods that affect your health—often in ways you may not even be aware of—and customizing your meals based on what's best for your body.

E Is for Ecological

Ecological eating is about being aware of where your food comes from—how it's sourced, grown, stored, and treated. By eating food from local sources, people can synergistically promote easier access to healthy, vibrant, fresh foods. Ideally, the environment should be enhanced, not destroyed, in the quest for good food.

If you have space for it, try growing your own food. If you live in an apartment, you can still easily grow herbs and greens in a sunny window—and your children will love helping with the planting and caretaking (especially if it involves making a mess with the dirt!). Growing your own food has the added benefits of an increased sense of purpose and regular outdoor time!

N Is for Nutritarian

I borrow this term from Dr. Joel Fuhrman, a family physician and best-selling nutritional researcher who wrote *Eat to Live*. Simply, a nutritarian diet consists of eating nutrient-dense food. This concept ties in with the ecological concerns discussed previously, because how food is farmed, and sometimes how it's cooked, affects its nutrient levels. One particularly memorable study I read analyzed the mineral content of spinach. The best spinach and the worst spinach, cooked or raw, had a 1,500-fold difference in their iron content. I'd much rather eat the iron-dense spinach than the depleted spinach! Part of the problem is you can't tell just by looking at the spinach whether it was grown locally in dense soil with naturally based fertilizers unless you speak to the farmer. The fresher the food, the more it retains its nutrients.

THE ENERGY-BOOSTING EATING PLAN

As you learned in chapter 5, the best way you can eat to tackle your postnatal depletion is by eating a diet with fats, protein, and carbohydrates in a ratio that will, for most, be different from how you were previously eating. This means higher levels of fats, moderate levels of protein, and low levels of carbohydrates.

Your diet should consist of an ideal ratio of around 20 to 25 percent of caloric (or energy) intake from protein, 50 to 60 percent of caloric intake from fats, and 20 to 30 percent of caloric intake from carbohydrates. No, these numbers aren't wrong—this is simply a different way to eat when you're depleted! But it helps to understand that there is a lot of fat in food that we may not necessarily suspect, and fat is much more energy dense than carbohydrates, and it is found in foods such as fish, nuts, and seeds. A gram of fat has about the same energy as 3 g carbohydrates.

To truly reduce inflammation and get the full benefits of this dietary ratio, you should stick with it for at least six weeks. Many mothers feel benefits within a week, but our goal is not just to *feel* better but to *be* better as well. And this takes a bit of time.

Once you have changed how you eat, you'll have a much clearer idea after six weeks about which foods are and are not your friends. Your system will be much cleaner, and you will have eliminated many triggers, so when you reintroduce different foods you'll quickly know what makes you particularly tired, brain fogged, or bloated. I find that most of my mothers feel so much better after six weeks on this eating plan that they have no desire to go back to eating grains the way they used to. Many mothers express an initial hesitation when I first show them this food plan, but they quickly adjust and are thrilled with the results.

How Often to Eat

Most depleted mothers need three meals per day, but once their depletion is healed, some do well with only two meals per day. There's no golden rule—just guidelines. Breakfast is the most important meal of the day, so choose strategically. Once you are in the rhythm of the diet and your body is being restored and recovering, you'll find that your need to snack decreases, as do your cravings for sweets and salt.

Some of the Best Foods to Eat for Breakfast

- **Quinoa:** Add fresh fruit to quinoa while cooking, then top with dates, nuts, coconut oil, and maple syrup.
- **Baked eggs:** Bake eggs in a homemade tomato sauce with spinach, and top with dukka (1 teaspoon sesame seeds, 1 teaspoon coriander seeds, ½ teaspoon cumin seeds, 2 tablespoons toasted hazelnuts, salt, and pepper, whizzed together in a food processor or blender).
- **Breakfast bowl:** Blend together frozen berries, 1 frozen banana, 2 teaspoons chia seeds, cinnamon, powdered ginger, vanilla extract, yogurt of choice (sheep, goat, buffalo, and coconut are better than cow dairy), and 1 tablespoon maca powder. Top with cacao nibs, bee pollen, toasted nuts, and goji berries.
- **Sweet or savory pancakes:** Mix 1 cup almond meal, 1 teaspoon vanilla extract, cinnamon, and a pinch of salt into 2 beaten eggs, stir, and thin out a little with milk of choice. Fry into pancakes and serve topped with warm berries and maple syrup or smoked salmon, goat cheese, and fresh herbs.
- **Scrambled eggs:** Scramble eggs with pesto, and serve with bacon/ham or smoked fish, fresh tomato, and sauerkraut.
- **Revive green smoothie:** Blend together 2 cups coconut water, 1 tablespoon nut butter, 1 fresh/frozen banana, 1 tablespoon maca powder, 1 tablespoon spirulina, 1 generous handful of greens (e.g., spinach, kale, mint, parsley), and ½ teaspoon bee pollen.
- **Poached eggs:** Serve poached eggs with fried zucchini, goat cheese, and pesto.
- **Porridge:** Make porridge from oats, quinoa, millet, or amaranth, and serve with ground flaxseed, almonds, macadamias, cinnamon, coconut milk, and fresh berries.

Your Daily Ratio

You will likely be eating fewer carbs and sweets than you're used to. The lists following this section will give you lots of options for what's best to eat and to avoid. But you will be aiming for 20 to 25 percent protein, 50 to 60 percent fats, and 20 to 30 percent carbohydrates. You will need to modify based on what feels best for your body, but it's important to start with this balance and choose foods that work best for you.

Cooking Doesn't Have to Be a Chore!

For many of the mothers I see, cooking is a dreaded, uncreative chore, and they beat themselves up when they feel they are "underperforming" in this department. In an ideal world, we would be sourcing our food locally from fresh sources, enjoying a village-style shopping experience, and approaching the creation of meals with inspiration and pleasure. However, the reality is often a long way from here, with many depleted mothers describing to me their frustration and exhaustion around the seemingly never-ending cycle of shopping, cooking, and cleaning up.

My advice is *stop beating yourself up*. Don't compare yourself to anyone else. You are doing the best you can. If you are struggling, remember that the situation is only temporary and that as you start to address your micronutrient and macronutrient levels, you will feel less foggy and more energized. With increased energy comes heightened motivation and inspiration. Along with that, take heart in the knowledge that good, healthy food does not have to be complicated or elaborate to be delicious and nourishing.

New moms, saddled with low energy, baby brain, and/or cravings, sometimes tend to prioritize other, seemingly more urgent tasks over food preparation, which can lead to unhealthy, "easy" food choices. If this sounds like you, know that this is common and just start fresh again the next day. Once you start eating more fats it will help you with the consistency of your energy, which is like putting a slow-burning log on the fire that can sustain you for hours—as opposed to eating carbs, which is like putting on twigs that burn up immediately.

Reach out to your networks of support. Think about getting together with other parents and children to make food together to bring in an element of community spirit. Take a cooking class. Join or start a freezer party or meal-prep club, so you can swap food with others. Cooking and food preparation don't come naturally to everyone, and that's okay.

WELCOME TO SMOOTHIE WORLD

I am in charge of my family's smoothie making—this is a daily ritual. Both Caroline and I have a smoothie for breakfast every morning, and the kids usually have a small one alongside whatever else they might be eating, too. We make a batch, and whatever we don't drink at breakfast time is consumed later in the day.

For us, smoothies are the easiest and most delicious way to ingest some pretty powerful immune-boosting superfoods. Caroline swears this daily ritual is the reason why in the last few years our family does not seem as susceptible to sickness during cold and flu season.

Oscar's Smoothie Ingredients

I don't measure out exact quantities and I change around ingredients regularly. I make enough in the blender for our entire family. Have fun experimenting!

Take it easy on yourself and make simple meals that you and your children will enjoy. Find four to six nutritious meals that you can cook easily, and keep these on high rotation. Eat what your kids eat—you're creating a huge and unnecessary workload if you cook different or more sophisticated meals for yourself. Kids normally prefer colorful fresh meals, which is perfect for serving up nutrient-dense food for the whole family. Keep lots of ingredients in the pantry to add instant zing, crunch, and flavor, such as tamari, olive oil, lemons, nuts and seeds, tahini, pesto, and mustards. Even if only for the time being, be content to eat simply at home, and go out for fancier meals on date night with your partner.

Get in the habit of throwing together a filling salad with simple ingredients. Using a foundation of fresh greens, shoots, and raw grated veggies or cold leftover roasted veggies, add the yummy fats, protein, and extras: avocado, pine nuts, goat cheese, hard-boiled egg, capers, olives, cashews, tempeh, cold chicken, and bacon bits, drizzled all over with olive oil and lemon and sprinkled with salt and pepper to taste. This can be a quick-and-easy meal when you are hungry or tired.

- Coconut water or spring water
- Protein powder
- Cacao nibs, cacao butter, or cacao powder
- Chia seeds
- Frozen organic berries
- Banana or other seasonal fruit
- Maca powder or other superfood

Some of the Best Foods to Eat for Lunch and Dinner

The foods in the following list are rich in all the micronutrients and macronutrients mentioned in the previous chapters, plus they're a great source of antioxidants and bioflavonoids. Bioflavonoids are the colorful pigments in foods that help reduce inflammation in the body.

If you're used to eating sandwiches, substitute large salads with a lot of different veggies and a warm protein such as chicken breast or fish. You'll be so full you won't miss the bread at all! I also like stir-fries with brown basmati rice, veggies, and protein.

- Mexican Bowl of Joy: organic corn chips, beans (kidney/adzuki), Yummy Tomato Sauce (see page 155), shredded lettuce, avocado slices, and a generous squeeze of lime.
- Poached fish or a can of sardines/mackerel, warmed, served with hard-boiled egg and steamed sweet potato and greens. Drizzle with oil, lemon, and fresh herbs/sesame seeds.

- Fried lamb patties (minced lamb, fresh ginger, paprika, ground cumin, and beaten egg) served with salad greens, cucumber, and Yummy Tomato Sauce (see page 155) or yogurt.
- Sliced cooked chicken served with a salad of red bell pepper, carrot, greens, mint, and papaya; dressing for salad: apple cider vinegar, honey, lime, and coconut oil.
- Liver fried in sesame or olive oil with ginger, garlic, spinach, red bell peppers, and a good splash of tamari.
- Roasted sweet potato drizzled with sesame oil and served with avocado and nut butter.
- Buckwheat noodles cooked and then fried in ginger, garlic, and sesame oil and served with steamed broccoli and salmon. Season with tamari or Yummy Lemon Pine Nut Dressing: ¼ cup toasted pine nuts, 1 scallion, 2 tablespoons fresh lemon juice, 2 tablespoons extra-virgin olive oil, pepper, and salt.
- Brown rice (soaked for 5 hours in filtered water, rinsed, and cooked) served with pan-fried fish, lemon, spinach, garlic, ginger, and coconut oil. Season with 1 tablespoon miso paste, thinned with a little boiling water.
- Chicken wraps: cooked chicken, salad greens, tomato, grated carrot, beet, avocado, and coconut mayonnaise wrapped in a spelt/whole-wheat/gluten-free wrap. For the coconut mayo, blend the flesh of 1 young coconut with garlic, lemon, sea salt, fresh herbs; slowly add 1½ teaspoons coconut water.
- Slow-cooked lamb shank served with cauliflower nut mash and bitter greens. For the mash, lightly steam the cauliflower, then mix in a food processor with macadamia nuts, garlic, and sea salt; slowly add 1 cup almond milk or coconut water. Also good with baked fish or chicken.
- Chicken soup: 1 whole raw chicken, sautéed red onion, garlic, ginger, vegetable/bone broth, veggies of choice, and 1 cut-up rinsed strip of kombu. Cook on low heat for 2 hours.
- Grilled salmon fillets served with salad greens, soft-boiled egg, cherry tomatoes, and asparagus; dressing: lemon, flax oil, and apple cider vinegar.

- Cooked dried Puy (French green) lentils or rinsed store-bought lentils from a BPA-free (bisphenol-A-free) can fried in olive oil with red onion, spices, veggies of choice, and a little bone broth and topped with goat cheese and fresh herbs.
- Zucchini pasta: Peel the zucchini into long strips with a potato peeler, then slice into thinner strips and combine with a splash of olive oil and fresh herbs. Serve with warmed Yummy Tomato Sauce and goat cheese.

For the Yummy Tomato Sauce, if you are lucky enough to live near a farmers' market, ask a tomato vendor if they have seconds. Rinse, core, slice, and cook in a saucepan over very low heat for about 2 hours, just in a little olive oil. Herbs, such as basil, oregano, thyme, tarragon, chives, or parsley, may be added if you like. (I like to make a big batch of it and freeze portion sizes so that it's always on hand.)

Some of the Best Foods to Eat for Snacks

You may need to snack between meals if you're breastfeeding or if you have blood sugar fluctuations (dizziness when standing, feeling faint when hungry, having mood swings when hungry). For some people, eating smaller meals more regularly is ideal; for others, sticking to three square meals per day is better, particularly if you have finished breastfeeding and are trying to lose weight. There's no right or wrong to this, as you know what your body prefers. (Remember, it is never advisable to try to lose any weight by minimizing calories while breastfeeding—you could be depriving your baby and yourself of much-needed nutrients.)

Best Healthy Snacks

- Hard-boiled eggs with a sprinkle of sea salt. Boil up a half dozen at the start of the week and keep in the fridge for a fast protein-packed snack.
- Bone broth.
- Chicken soup as a leftover snack.

- Vegetable sticks or leftover roasted veggies with homemade hummus. For the hummus, blend together a BPA-free can of chickpeas (or 1 cup soaked and cooked chickpeas), ¼ cup tahini, juice from ½ lemon, ¼ cup olive oil, 1 garlic clove, salt, and pepper. Add a little water to gain the consistency you like and adjust lemon juice, garlic, and seasonings to taste. Serve with slices of carrot, cucumber, peppers, and celery.
- A handful of mixed unsalted nuts.
- Tamari-roasted seeds. Take a mix of seeds, such as sunflower and pumpkin seeds, toss with a little tamari and coconut oil, and roast slowly at 325°F for 10 minutes. Give them a shake and roast for another 5 to 10 minutes, until golden. Keep them in an airtight container.

What to Drink

The very best thing you can drink is plain old water, preferably spring or filtered. When you're depleted, be sure to drink at least 64 ounces/8 cups every day. When you're breastfeeding, you should drink at least 80 ounces/10 cups every day.

Other Beneficial Drinks

- Herbal teas. A good source of hydration that contains health properties. Some herbs that are great and safe for nourishing moms include nettle, chamomile, holy basil, oat straw, and raspberry leaf. Rosehip and nettle tea is energizing and rich in minerals and vitamin C; add fresh ginger for a kick. Peppermint and lemon balm teas are helpful for digestion.
- Coffee and black tea. Coffee can be fine for some women but depleting for others. If coffee makes you feel buzzy or anxious, and if you are relying on it for energy, then it's probably best to wean yourself off it and switch to decaf or herbal teas. Black tea is a gentler alternative but can still have too much caffeine for some.

- Smoothies. A great choice and preferable to juices as they contain the fiber that slows down the rate at which natural sugars are absorbed and levels out your energy for longer periods. Adding protein and good fats to a smoothie will create a quick and easy meal or snack.
- Coconut water. Electrolyte rich and hydrating.
- Yummy hot cocoa. Mix together raw cacao, cinnamon, maca powder, and a dash of both ground cayenne and vanilla powder. Dissolve in boiled water and add heated milk of choice. Sweeten with a little honey or coconut sugar. This drink is strengthening, mineral rich, and fortifying.
- Small cup of bone broth. Rich in collagen in its denatured form, which makes it very easy to digest and absorb, bone broth is really good for you. About one-quarter of all of the protein in your body is collagen; it's like the scaffolding that all our tendons, ligaments, bones, and teeth need in order to maintain form and strength. It is vital for our skeletal and muscular health as well as the health of our digestive tract. A big part of the accelerated aging (sagging skin and hair loss) that mothers worry about is actually just collagen loss. The body can make collagen out of plant proteins, but bone broth is a faster, quicker way for this to happen—so drink up! If you make broth, you'll know you've cooked it long enough if it gels in the fridge overnight. I like to infuse mine with star anise or ginger for added flavor.
- Roasted dandelion root. Bring to a slow boil 1 to 2 tablespoons dandelion root, fresh or ground ginger and star anise, and 1 to 2 cups water. Simmer for 5 minutes. Serve with milk of choice and honey. This is mineral rich, alkalizing, supportive of the liver, and a good alternative to coffee.

THE BEST WAYS TO COOK TO PRESERVE NUTRIENTS

Steaming and baking are the best ways to preserve nutrients by cooking. Steam for the minimal amount of time allowed so that the vegetable is cooked but still has a healthy texture and bright color. Because boiling causes valuable nutrients to leach into the cooking water, I avoid this method.

As for microwaves, there is a lot of contradictory advice when it comes to their safety, so I recommend using them only to heat up food in glass containers. This way, you maintain the nutrients and enzymes within the food, especially breast milk, and there is no leaching of known harmful plastics into the food. If, on the other hand, you use a microwave to cook food from start to finish in nonglass containers, you risk losing nutrients, destroying enzymes, and introducing harmful plastic residues in your food. A better choice for quickly heating up food and for cooking is a steam convection oven.

Two Days of Family Meals

Day 1

Breakfast

Porridge (see page 150)

Lunch

Sliced cooked chicken (see page 154)

Dinner

Buckwheat noodles (see page 154)

Snacks

Revive green smoothie (see page 150)
Square of dark chocolate
Mixed unsalted nuts
Fruit
Cocoa with cinnamon

Day 2

Breakfast

Scrambled eggs with pesto (see page 150)

Lunch

Mexican Bowl of Joy (see page 153)

Dinner

Slow-cooked lamb shank (see page 154)

Snacks

Fresh ginger tea infused with lemon balm, nettle, and hibiscus
Miso soup with rice noodles
Vegetable sticks with hummus (see page 155)
Berries with sheep/goat yogurt and ground flaxseed

Sample Seven-Day Meal Plan

Seven Days of Breakfast

- Berry and cacao butter smoothie
- Big breakfast: Bacon and eggs with spinach, zucchini, mushrooms, and avocado
- Chia pudding with coconut yogurt and fruits
- Mushroom omelet with smoked salmon on the side
- Paleo muesli with coconut yogurt and berries
- Pancakes (see page 150)
- Porridge (see page 150)

Seven Days of Lunch

- Sashimi or sushi
- Chicken breast with cashew salad
- Smoked salmon and eggs and avocado
- Gado-gado—eggs, tempeh, salad, satay sauce
- Rice-paper rolls with egg and tempeh
- Chicken soup (see page 154)
- Frittata
- Niçoise salad

Seven Days of Dinner

- Paleo butter chicken and salad
- Burgers and salad
- Baked fish with lemon butter and veggies/salad
- Zucchini pasta (see page 155)
- Steak and veggies
- Blue-corn tortilla with guacamole and beans and chicken or ground beef
- A "family roast" of chicken, lamb, or beef with roasted vegetables

Shopping List

Always buy organic when possible.

Fats

- ☑ Coconut oil
- ☑ Cold-pressed olive oil
- ☑ Cold-pressed walnut oil
- ☑ Ghee

Protein

- ☑ Beans, canned or dried—kidney, black, chickpeas, cannellini
- ☑ Free-range chicken
- ☑ Free-range eggs
- ☑ Fresh fish
- ☑ Ham or bacon
- ☑ Hummus
- ☑ Minced lamb or grass-fed beef
- ☑ Mixed nuts—almonds, macadamia, walnut
- ☑ Nut butters
- ☑ Smoked fish

Grains

- ☑ Buckwheat noodles
- ☑ Millet, hulled
- ☑ Oats, rolled (not quick cooking)
- ☑ Quinoa
- ☑ Rice noodles

Dairy

- ☑ Butter
- ☑ Goat cheese
- ☑ Sheep or goat yogurt

Vegetables

- ☑ Avocado
- ☑ Cauliflower
- ☑ Cucumber
- ☑ Herbs, fresh (mint, parsley, cilantro, etc.)
- ☑ Mixed greens
- ☑ Red bell pepper
- ☑ Tomato
- ☑ Zucchini

Fruits

- ☑ Apples
- ☑ Bananas
- ☑ Berries, fresh or frozen
- ☑ Citrus
- ☑ Other seasonal fruits

Other

- ☑ Almond milk
- ☑ Apple cider vinegar
- ☑ Cocoa, cold-pressed
- ☑ Coconut milk
- ☑ Coconut water
- ☑ Collagen or protein powder
- ☑ Corn chips
- ☑ Dandelion root, roasted
- ☑ Dark chocolate
- ☑ Goji berries
- ☑ Ground flaxseed (or buy fresh and grind your own in a blender for freshness; store in the fridge)
- ☑ Himalayan salt
- ☑ Honey
- ☑ Miso soup packets
- ☑ Pesto
- ☑ Rice or corn cakes
- ☑ Sauerkraut
- ☑ Spirulina, dried
- ☑ Teas: dried nettle, hibiscus, lemon balm

CHOOSING NUTRIENT-DENSE FRUITS AND VEGETABLES

Research by Jo Robinson, author of *Eating on the Wild Side*, and many others has shown how nutrient content differs among varieties of plants and how methods of spraying, ripening, harvesting, and storage can affect nutrients, too. The fewer nutrients you lose from your food, the better that food will be for your body and the better you'll feel.

One of the consequences of cultivating the sweetest and mildest-tasting wild plants over generations has been a dramatic loss of nutrients. Heirloom varieties of fruits and vegetables are more nutrient dense than their hybrid counterparts. Modern produce is bred to be sturdy for transport and disease resistant, and it generally contains higher levels of sugar. Many of the most beneficial antioxidants and nutrients have a sour, astringent, or bitter taste, but these are being bred out of our foods.

In addition, it is believed that the principal reason that humans see color the way that we do is so we can correctly identify the ripest and most nutrient- and antioxidant-rich fruits and vegetables. The best antioxidants are, in fact, the "pigments" that give these plants their bright, vivid colors. It is no accident that we are attracted to colorful food, and it brings new meaning to the idea of "eating the rainbow."

Allium Family

Alliums include garlic, onions, shallots, leeks, scallions, and chives.

Did you know that three cloves of garlic contain the same antibacterial activity as a standard dose of penicillin? Well, they do! Garlic truly is a superfood. Chop, mince, or slice garlic and leave it away from the heat for ten minutes. During this time the maximum amount of allicin, the active antibacterial agent, will be formed.

When buying onions, look for firm ones with an intact outer skin. There is a high concentration of nutrients in onion skins, so save them and add to soup broths. Pouring a teaspoon of vinegar on the surface of your cutting board before you start to chop onions will alleviate tearing eyes.

Shallots are superstars of the allium family, containing six times more nutrients than onions.

With leeks, the most nutrients are in the stalk. Buy small ones with tender stalks, and cook them as soon as possible because they quickly lose antioxidant benefits.

Apples

The highest concentration of antioxidants and nutrients is found in the skin, so always eat it! But because apple skins also contain the highest level of pesticide residue of any fruit or vegetable, buy organic apples only. Apples are stored best in the fridge.

Artichokes, Asparagus, and Avocados

Artichokes, asparagus, and avocados all are rich in antioxidants, nutrients, and fiber and low in sugar. It's hard to go wrong with them, which is why I love the nickname the A Team.

Because artichokes have a high antioxidant content, they need to be as fresh as possible. Use them quickly, as these levels can significantly drop within seven to ten days. Paradoxically, boiling artichokes increases their antioxidant levels, but steaming is even better. Although fresh is best, frozen or canned artichokes still contain considerable amounts of antioxidants.

As with artichokes, asparagus is best fresh, and cooked asparagus has more antioxidants than raw. Steaming is the way to go.

Avocados are an excellent source of soluble fiber and good fats, with the Hass variety being the most nutrient dense.

Berries

All berries are high in antioxidants, vitamin C, and anthocyanins (the latter have a powerful anti-inflammatory effect). They have a low glycemic index (sugar load) and are rich in fiber, too. Because berries spoil quickly, they should be eaten immediately or put in the fridge for no more than three days.

Frozen berries are almost as nutritious as fresh berries. Thawing in the microwave is best for retaining nutrient levels. Cooked or canned blueberries can have greater antioxidant levels than fresh blueberries.

Carrots

Purple carrots are more nutritious than orange due to high levels of the bioflavonoid anthocyanin. Cooked carrots are more nutritious than raw. Include some fats or oil with the meal. Steaming or baking whole carrots preserves more of their nutrients.

Citrus Fruits

The deeper the color of citrus, the more antioxidants and nutrient content. Citrus fruits can be kept on the kitchen counter for a week but should be put in the fridge for longer storage.

Navel oranges are popular and nutritious. Go for the largest with uniform, deep orange color and juiciness.

Red and pink grapefruit are sweeter tasting than white grapefruit.

Corn

Choose non-GMO corn or heirloom varieties, and bake or steam with the husks on. Avoid supersweet corn, as it has low levels of protein and high levels of sugar.

Cruciferous Vegetables

Cruciferous veggies—broccoli, cabbage, cauliflower, and Brussels sprouts—are high in glucosinolates, sulfur-containing nutrients that assist with immune function. All crucifers are also rich in antioxidants.

Eat broccoli that is as fresh as possible. Ten days after harvest, broccoli loses more than 80 percent of its glucosinolates, 75 percent of its flavonoids, and 50 percent of its vitamin C. To preserve nutrients, broccoli must be chilled as soon as it is harvested, kept cool, and then eaten within two to three days. Store it in a microperforated bag; place your green leafy vegetables or your cruciferous vegetables in a resealable plastic bag, squeeze out the air, seal the bag, and use a needle or pin to prick between ten and twenty evenly spaced holes. Store it in the crisper of your fridge for twice the antioxidant activity. Steaming for four minutes is the best way to retain nutrients and prevents the formation of unpleasant odors and flavors.

Cabbage can be stored for weeks longer than other cruciferous veggies without losing nutrients.

White cauliflower is best steamed or sautéed to maintain nutrients.

Grapes/Raisins

Red, purple, and black grapes are best for your health. The best varieties are red flame and black seedless. Go organic.

Legumes

Legumes are high in protein but low in the amino acid methionine, which is necessary to form a high-quality, more complete protein. Most grains are rich in methionine but lack the other essential amino acids that legumes have in spades. When grains and legumes are eaten together, a complete protein is formed that is of the same quality as that found in meat, eggs, and dairy products.

All dried peas and beans are high in soluble fiber, antioxidants, and nutrients. If you soak dried beans overnight, you can reduce their intestinal gaseous effect; be sure to discard the soaking liquid, rinse them well, and cook in fresh water. Dried beans can also be cooked in a pressure cooker, which is a great way to retain the most antioxidant activity.

Canned peas and beans lose much of their flavor and nutritional value; studies show that canning peas destroys 50 percent of their antioxidants. Freezing green beans and peas, on the other hand, destroys only about 25 percent. Interestingly, canned kidney beans and pinto beans retain more nutrients and antioxidants than do other canned legumes.

Potatoes

New potatoes do not raise your blood sugar as much as mature potatoes do, and organic is always best. In addition to eating the skins, you can lower the glycemic index of potatoes by eating them with fat. Chilling potatoes for twenty-four hours after they've been cooked changes their starch to a more beneficial form, which is very healthy for your gut bacteria.

Salad Greens

The most nutritious greens are intensely colored reds, purples, and reddish browns, which contain the highest levels of antioxidants, nutrients, and anti-inflammatory anthocyanins. When the leaves are loose and open they produce more antioxidants and nutrients as part of the plant's own "sunscreen" production. The more tightly wrapped the leaves of a leafy vegetable (like a cabbage or iceberg lettuce), the lower the nutrient levels.

The fresher the better, so opt for whole lettuce rather than precut. To store, pull off the leaves, rinse them, and soak for ten minutes in very cold water. The cold water slows the aging process by increasing internal moisture. Dry with a tea towel or salad spinner.

If you tear up the lettuce before you store it, you can double its antioxidant value. The living plant responds self-protectively to the insult, as if it were being gnawed by an insect or eaten by an animal, and produces a burst of antioxidants and nutrients to fend off the intruders. However, lettuce should be stored torn only if it will be eaten within a day or two, because tearing the leaves also hastens decay.

Other preserving tips: Store the greens in a resealable plastic bag, squeeze out the air, seal the bag, and use a needle or pin to prick between ten and twenty evenly spaced holes. Store the bag in the crisper drawer of your fridge. This allows for gases and moisture to escape. Let the greens breathe!

Look for deeply colored, wide-leaf varieties of these nutritious salad greens:

- Arugula: This member of the cabbage family is high in antioxidants such as glucosinolates and is also higher in calcium, magnesium, folate, and vitamin E than most other salad greens are.
- Radicchio: The best variety of this member of the chicory family is Italian Rosso di Chioggia, which is loose leaf, red, and

bitter. Radicchio is high in B-group vitamins and vitamin C as well as minerals, polyphenols (which include health-promoting antioxidants), and probiotics.

- Spinach: Spinach is best steamed; do not boil or the nutrients will be leached into the cooking water.
- Wild greens, such as dandelion leaves and beet greens, have high levels of nutrients, including calcium.

Make sure your salad dressing includes a healthy fat, such as extra-virgin olive oil, as it makes the nutrients more bioavailable.

Enrich your lettuce choice with other varieties of greens. You can tame the bold flavor of bitter greens by adding fruit or avocado to the salad or honey to the dressing.

Stone Fruits

Peaches and nectarines are identical except for one gene that codes for fuzziness and a few other minor traits. The skin is the most nutritious part but also susceptible to pesticide residue, so choose organic fruits when possible.

Freezing preserves more antioxidants than canning does. To preserve the most antioxidant activity when freezing, first slice the fruit and sprinkle it with powdered vitamin C.

The queen of the dried fruits is prunes, which are dried plums. Buy them sulfite-free (sulfites are a preservative you don't need). They are high in antioxidants, soluble and insoluble fiber, and sorbitol, a prebiotic that promotes healthy gut microbes and regular bowels.

Tomatoes

Tomatoes produce lycopene to protect themselves from UV rays. Lycopene is an antioxidant particularly useful in helping the body repair damaged tissues. Processed tomatoes are surprisingly nutritious. Buy them in cans that are BPA-free or in glass.

Tomato paste, the most concentrated form of processed tomato, has up to ten times more lycopene than raw tomatoes.

Tropical Fruits

Bananas are relatively low in nutrients and they have a high glycemic load, so they shouldn't be eaten that often.

Guavas have a higher nutrient density than other tropical fruits.

Mangoes have five times more vitamin C than oranges, five times more fiber than pineapples, and a moderate glycemic load. Darker varieties have the most phytonutrients.

Papaya has a very low glycemic load and is an excellent source of vitamin C. Red flesh is more nutritious than yellow.

With pineapples, sweeter is better, as these varieties have more beta-carotene and vitamin C.

THE BEST FOODS AND SUPERFOODS

This is a go-to list of foods that tend to be higher in nutrients and antioxidants and lower in inflammation-causing proteins.

Carbohydrates

- Amaranth
- Buckwheat
- Freekeh
- Fruits
- Kamut
- Legumes (lentils, beans, and chickpeas)
- Millet
- Oats
- Quinoa, chia seeds, and hemp seeds
- Rice (brown, red, black, basmati, jasmine)
- Vegetables

Fats

- Avocado and avocado oil
- Butter
- Coconut oil
- Hemp seed oil
- Ghee
- Nuts, nut butters, and nut oils
- Olive oil

Protein

Animal Sources (preferably organic and free-range)

- Beef
- Chicken
- Eggs
- Fish
- Full-fat goat, sheep, or cow dairy (milk, cheese, unsweetened yogurt, cream)
- Lamb
- Seafood

Plant Sources

- Chia seeds
- Hemp seeds
- Legumes (lentils, beans, and chickpeas)
- Quinoa

Other

- Herbs: basil, cilantro, parsley, rosemary, tarragon, and thyme
- Aromatics: chiles, garlic, galangal, and ginger
- Spices: anise, cardamom, caraway, cinnamon, coriander, cumin, paprika, pepper, sumac, and turmeric

Superfoods

- Berries: high in antioxidants, vitamin C, and fiber; low glycemic level
- Cacao and dark chocolate: high in magnesium, iron, manganese, and antioxidants (look for those with 75 percent or more cocoa solids)
- Chia: high in omega-3s, antioxidants, fiber, and calcium; good carb and protein source
- Dandelion root tea or coffee: gently supportive of the liver and helpful in the detoxification of hormones
- Green tea: high in antioxidants
- Maca: supportive of energy production, hormone balancing, thyroid health, and your body as a whole in times of stress
- Seeds (pumpkin, sunflower, hemp): high in fiber and healthy fats; nutrient dense

Sugar Alternatives

All sweeteners should be used in small amounts. Try to avoid all sugars listed on pages 172–173 and replace them with small amounts of the following. Health foods stores should stock all of these.

- Artichoke syrup
- Coconut sugar
- Lacuma powder
- Pure maple syrup
- Molasses
- Raw honey
- Stevia

You can naturally sweeten baked goods and homemade snacks with dried fruits such as dates or with applesauce.

Foods Rich in Micronutrients

Copper

Organ meats, cacao, seeds, nuts

Iron

Red meat, dark green leafy vegetables, beans and legumes, seafood, poultry

Magnesium

Green leafy vegetables, cacao, seeds, nuts, legumes

Trace Elements, Including Iodine and Selenium

All foods, especially sea vegetables and superfoods

Vitamin B_{12}

Fermented foods like kefir, sauerkraut, and miso; algae, eggs, mushrooms, red meat, seafood, dairy

Other B vitamins

All foods, especially green leafy vegetables and most fruits (the amount depends on the quality of the food, how it was grown, and how fresh it is)

Vitamin C

Citrus fruits, all berries

Vitamin D

Fortified milk, organ meats, cod liver oil; small amounts in mushrooms, eggs

Fat-Soluble Vitamins, Especially Vitamins K_2 and A

For vitamin A: colorful vegetables such as carrots, cod liver oil, dairy, eggs

For vitamin E: animal fats such as butter, avocado, nuts, some seeds

For vitamin K_2: aged cheeses; eggs, especially free-range and pasture-raised eggs (two eggs a day is enough to maintain vitamin K_2 levels); fermented dairy such as kefir; fermented foods such as miso, *nattō* (Japanese fermented soybeans), tempeh

Zinc

Shellfish, red meat, chicken, eggs, dairy, legumes, nuts, seeds, grains

FOOD AND DRINK TO AVOID

In General

There are many food groups that postnatally depleted women need to reduce or avoid on their path to recovery. Basically, the only kind of food your body knows how to digest is *real*, unprocessed food. Eating "fake" foods, such as potato chips, microwave pizza, or sweetened drinks, which have been concocted in test kitchens to trick your taste buds, is like putting water into your gas tank. It won't keep you running and is only going to confuse your body.

Instead, aiming for nutrient-dense foods will provide you with energy while supporting a healthy body and mind. Time to toss the fake foods out of your pantry!

Carbohydrates

Carbohydrates are found naturally in vegetables, fruit, legumes, and whole grains and are meant to be broken down slowly so that energy is released gradually and beneficial nutrients are absorbed. Processed carbohydrates have had the nutrients removed and can spike our blood sugar levels too quickly; they are also difficult for our digestive systems to process.

Where Processed Carbohydrates Are Found

- Baked goods made with white flour, sugar, and/or trans fats
- Breads, including white bread and gluten-free breads made from processed gluten-free grains

- Candy
- Frosting from a can
- Pasta made from white flour
- Potato chips and pretzels
- Rice cakes
- Sugar
- White flours

Fats

Synthetic trans fats are found in the partially hydrogenated vegetable oils often used in baked and fried goods. They promote inflammation, depress the immune system, and have been linked to reproductive disorders, heart disease and stroke, cancers, and diabetes. Avoid the following (and swap for healthy options from "The Best Foods and Superfoods" section on page 168):

- Canola oil
- Chips
- Corn oil
- Crackers
- Deep-fried foods
- French fries
- Margarine
- Peanut oil

Protein

Processed meats, seafood, and dairy usually contain a host of manmade ingredients that are not great for our health. Deli meats such as ham, bacon, and chicken are commonly injected with preservatives to prolong shelf life, and nonorganic meats and eggs can contain synthetic hormones and antibiotics that have been given to the animals as they are raised or residues from stock feed, some of which have been found to include animal by-products, urea, and arsenic compounds. The

AVOID FISH WITH HIGH MERCURY LEVELS

Mercury affects people differently, and there are different types of mercury found in different parts of the body with differing effects. How's that for different? And worrying! The most dangerous type of mercury is inorganic mercury, from industrial sources and amalgams used to fill your cavities, and methyl mercury, typically found in animal products and certain fish.

Your body has a limited ability to excrete heavy metals such as mercury, and it needs copious amounts of zinc and selenium to slowly do this. Of the many effects of mercury, it is the neurodevelopmental impact on young children that I am most worried about. If mercury were the only issue these

U.S. Department of Agriculture has strict restrictions on organic livestock and eggs to ensure they do not contain these potentially health-disrupting factors. Avoid the following:

- Nitrogen-preserved deli meats and bacon. Local farmers' markets and specialty grocers may have nitrogen-free options.
- Caged eggs. Aim to source eggs from local markets, and choose pasture-raised or organic varieties where possible.
- Processed cheese and dairy in which ingredients are not limited to milk, cream, salt, rennet, natural enzymes, and cultures. Avoid dairy products with preservatives, added colors and flavors, concentrates, or acids. Yogurt should not contain sugar or artificial sweeteners. Avoid low-fat dairy.
- Meat and poultry that isn't organic. Grass-fed is another good alternative.
- Farmed fish. Fish should be fresh and locally sourced where possible if waters are clean. Farmed fish, although improving in quality, can be subjected to the same antibiotics, growth hormones, and poor food sources as conventionally farmed meat.

young brains had to deal with, it would be less alarming—but combine mercury exposure with the high levels of air pollution in cities, a diet low in omega-3 fatty acids and high in oxidized, plant-based omega-6 fatty acids, and the results can be alarming.

To avoid food-based mercury, I never eat fish with very high mercury levels (very large fish such as swordfish, all species of shark, marlin, and albacore tuna), and you shouldn't eat it either. Also avoid fish that have moderate mercury levels and are low in selenium (shark, flake, sole), as this compounds the mercury effects. Take a 200 mcg tablet of selenium every time you eat a moderate-mercury fish to reduce the amount of mercury you absorb.

ADDITIVES, ENHANCERS, PRESERVATIVES, AND NONFOOD INGREDIENTS

Pick up a packaged food these days and it's hard not to see numbers and words that you need a chemistry degree to decipher. These are man-made chemicals that your body can't recognize—we're designed to consume, digest, and utilize foods in their natural forms in order to function at our best. Everything else just causes confusion and chaos with our cells. In fact, I see these additives as having a negative effect on mental functioning, especially on motivation and mental clarity due to inflammation. If you've been working to heal from depletion, you should know that overconsumption of these food additives is a giant step backward on your path to wellness. Here's what to avoid:

- Additives, preservatives, and colors. If an ingredient name contains numbers (e.g., preservative E211, color E104), then it's a chemical or fake-food substance your body won't recognize.
- Monosodium glutamate (MSG) and flavor enhancers. Look for and avoid flavor enhancers, MSG, and the additive numbers 627, 631, and 635.

- Artificial sweeteners. Anything labeled "diet" or "sugar-free" will contain aspartame, acesulfame potassium, sucralose, or saccharin, which are artificial sweeteners that are even worse for your health than sugar.
- Fake anything, including whipped cream from a can, for example, or fake cheese that contains modified oils and starches. Cheese should be made from milk, cream, salt, rennet, natural enzymes, and starter cultures. Period.
- Junk food and fast food. You know what I'm talking about.
- Packaged, precooked meals. If you do opt for these on the rare occasion, then always check the ingredients and avoid any fake ingredients mentioned in this list.
- Low-fat diet foods. These usually contain artificial flavors, fillers, and sugars that make up for the lack of flavor and texture once fat is removed.

Artificial Colors and Flavors

Artificial colors are made from chemicals derived from petroleum and can be neuroexcitatory, overstimulating receptors in certain areas of your brain. In 2007, a landmark study was published in the *Lancet* that showed a relationship between increased hyperactivity in children and many of the food additives in the following list. In England, many of these artificial colors were banned, but the same companies with the same products in Australia left these food additives in. They're often in foods sold in America, too.

Artificial flavors are also made from chemicals, but because these formulas are highly proprietary to the food companies that create and use them, the actual chemicals are not disclosed to consumers. Fake flavors, like fake colors, can negatively affect your brain, and they act directly on the glutamate system (glutamate is a neurotransmitter), which puts your brain in an agitated or overly alert state. Not surprisingly, one of the side effects of MSG consumption is insomnia. Concerning, too, is possible low-grade neuron damage that seems to be related to repeated MSG exposure. Fortunately, due to consumer complaints about headaches, flushing, sweating, and insomnia, MSG is being used much less now in American packaged foods than it used to be.

Always use natural flavors when possible in your cooking. Real vanilla extract tastes so much better than fake vanilla, and you need much less of it. Fake maple syrup is nothing but chemical-laden sugar of the worst kind—high-fructose corn syrup—so buy only pure maple syrup. And if the soy sauce you've pulled off the grocery shelf doesn't contain actual soybeans, put it back.

Food Additives to Avoid

Colors: 102, 104, 110, 122, 124, 129
Preservatives: 211, 220, 250, 280, 281, 282
Flavor enhancers (including MSG): 621, 627, 631, 635
Artificial sweeteners (found in all "diet" products): 951, 952, 954, 1201

Drinks

Our main source of liquid replenishment should always be water. Avoid these:

- Coffee drinks. They usually contain lots of added milk and sugar.
- Energy drinks. These are high in sugar, caffeine, and additives.
- Juice drinks. If made from concentrates or with added sugar or other additives, stay away from them. Cold-pressed or freshly squeezed vegetable or fruit juice with a meal is okay.
- Power drinks and shakes. These are high in sugar and additives.
- Protein drinks and shakes made from dairy whey protein. These tend to be inflammatory.
- Soda, regular and diet. Many of the moms I treat are addicted to soda, both diet and regular. Soda is truly a terrible thing: a regular 12-ounce can contains up to 12 teaspoons junk sugar. Diet sodas might not have any calories, but your body will still respond to the artificial sugar by releasing insulin. This is why so many people who drink diet soda can't lose weight. In addition,

many sodas have high levels of caffeine, sodium, acid (which rots your teeth), and preservatives. An ideal way to wean yourself off soda is to drink water with lemon slices in it or unsweetened herbal iced tea. Or get a SodaStream or other device that turns flat spring water into carbonated seltzer—but avoid the SodaStream flavor packets, as they are full of sugar and chemicals.

- Vitamin-enriched drinks. These don't contain vitamins in an amount that will improve your health. Your nutrients and vitamins should all come from real food.

Genetically Modified Foods

GMO stands for genetically modified organism, and the safety of GMO foods is a highly contentious and controversial issue. The American Academy of Environmental Medicine's position paper in May 2009 stated that "several animal studies indicate serious health risks associated with GMO food," including infertility, immune problems, accelerated aging, insulin regulation, and changes in major organs and the gastrointestinal system. Organic food should not contain any GMOs. For guidance, go to http://www.nongmoshoppingguide.com/.

Nonfiltered Tap Water

Spring water from a genuine source, packaged in recyclable glass, is the ideal drinking water. Straight tap water may contain chlorine and can interfere with your body's utilization of iodine, which then can have a harmful impact on thyroid health. You can call your local water board to find out what's in your water.

DEALING WITH FOOD INTOLERANCE

If your energy is lacking, if you've always had trouble losing weight and keeping it off, and if you're wondering if what you're eating could be the culprit, you may be intolerant or allergic to certain foods; the most common culprits are gluten and dairy.

KRYPTONITE FOODS YOU THINK ARE GOOD FOR YOU BUT ARE NOT

There are three categories of food that certain bodies simply do not tolerate to one degree or another. In honor of my superhero-loving children, we can call these energy zappers Kryptonite foods.

- Kryptonite Foods Type 1 manifest as an *allergic reaction*. Eat one of these foods and you will have a direct and immediate immune response.
- Kryptonite Foods Type 2 manifest as *food sensitivity*. Foods in this group cause less extreme, and often delayed, reactions from your immune system that typically take place at some point after you eat—this is why they can be so hard to diagnose. This may include joint pains, lethargy, or a headache hours or even days after eating the offending food.
- Kryptonite Foods Type 3 manifest as *food intolerance*, in which particular foods can't be fully digested. These foods will negatively affect your well-being, though they won't trigger an immune-system response. Lactose intolerance is a good example of this.
- Even though it can often take time to discover your individual Kryptonite foods, the search is always worthwhile. Learning to avoid your food triggers is like releasing a hand brake that was invisibly activated in your body. When that happens, you suddenly feel so much better that you honestly can't believe that not eating one kind of food could have such a potent effect on your energy and well-being.

Gluten

Did you know that the only mammals that can easily digest gluten are animals like rodents? Gluten intolerance is both the most common and the least understood food problem. Gluten is nature's preservative/protectant and is actually classified as a plant toxin. Humans derive no nutritional value from eating gluten—it's like the Styrofoam box that the nutritional part of the grain comes with. Because gluten is so hard to digest (bacteria have a hard time digesting it, too!), it is used as a preservative, filler, or texturizer (in sausages, for instance) and is even found in the pill capsules you swallow.

As the word suggests, gluten is glutinous and is a sticky, hard-to-digest protein produced by wheat (or other grasses) as a way of protecting itself from environmental damage from the sun; excessive moisture or dryness, heat, or cold; and insect or bacterial attack. The larger the size of the wheat grain, the more gluten the plant must produce to keep it stable. Centuries-old forms of wheat like spelt or Kamut have smaller grains, thus lower amounts of gluten. Traditional societies ferment their wheat—using sourdough starters, for example—for days and even weeks, which removes much of the gluten from the dough. Modern wheat used in Australia and North America, on the other hand, has been created to contain very large amounts of gluten.

Celiac disease is an autoimmune disease triggered by gluten in genetically susceptible individuals. It can cause serious health issues, including digestive issues, inflammation, growth restriction, lethargy and brain fog, and the growth of tumors. Genuine gluten intolerance, on the other hand, is a reaction to gluten that doesn't involve your immune system. Typically, it causes abdominal pain, nausea, and diarrhea.

The main issue with gluten is understanding how *your* body reacts to eating it. Eating small or moderate amounts of wheat and other grains every day may not affect you the way consuming large amounts would. If you find that you need to eliminate wheat gluten from your diet, be forewarned that its replacements typically contain rice flour, tapioca starch, and other simple carbohydrates that can spike your blood sugar, are often more calorie dense, and, on average, are much more expensive. Label reading is a must!

Dairy

Dairy is what I call a spectrum food that can range from junk food (sweetened low-fat yogurt) to a superfood (organic cultured butter). What usually causes abdominal symptoms after eating dairy is an intolerance to lactose, or milk sugar. This is due to an insufficient level of lactase, the enzyme that breaks down lactose. Levels of lactase can drop during pregnancy and so mild symptoms can become moderate symptoms. Mothers often become more aware of an underlying lactose intolerance during and after pregnancy and will experience bloating, gas, and stomachaches after eating dairy. It is the casein protein in dairy that is usually responsible for triggering sinus issues, skin problems such as eczema, lethargy, irritability, and brain fog.

The easiest and most practical way to test for a food intolerance is with a two-week elimination challenge. Any food can be challenged, but only one at a time, and there can be absolutely no slipups or you'll have to start all over again. I've found that if exhaustion or gut problems are an issue, eliminating gluten from the diet is a good starting point; if allergies and skin conditions are the main concern, then dairy should be eliminated first.

You may or may not feel an improvement in your symptoms during these two weeks—but that's not your goal. It's what happens in the twenty-four hours after your reexposure to the potentially offending food that's the test. When reintroducing the food, eat only a moderate amount of it; when retesting your gluten tolerance, for example, eat two slices of toast, not more. And try to do this on a day when you know you're not going to be affected by a lot of other stressors as well, as some people experience an exaggerated reaction that they'd never get otherwise from eating that food every day. Pay close attention to how you feel: the symptoms you may experience can include anything from headaches and body aches to skin breakouts, stiff joints, and moodiness. Don't worry—these symptoms quickly go away.

This test is usually pretty accurate after the first go, but if you're still not sure, you can repeat it two or three more times to be certain. To get the full benefits, a full six weeks is required. If you do have a positive reaction, then avoid that food completely until you have been feeling fantastic for some time. It's important to know that a food intolerance is not a sentence for life. Typically, after six to eighteen months, you might have an incidental exposure without any of the reaction you had after the first food challenge. In my experience with my patients, I hardly ever see anyone going back or even *wanting* to go back to that offending food, especially when they know how badly it makes them feel. Patients' primary struggle seems to occur during the first six weeks while they become accustomed to reading food labels, reevaluate where to shop and what to shop for, and find the motivation. But these experiences can be so profound that they are a positive, lasting way to change your relationship with food.

For moms who want more information on these topics, I recommend *Clean Gut* by cardiologist Alejandro Junger and *Grain Brain* by neurologist David Perlmutter.

Serena's Story

Serena saw me for a few visits when she was thirty-seven and her baby was eight months old. She'd always been a high achiever and was very distressed that her energy had plummeted since the birth of her child and was getting worse. She'd wake up zombie-like and found it hard to get going. By 9:00 p.m. she'd sleep "like the dead." She was craving coffee, was sensitive to bright lights and loud noises, and often got dizzy when she stood up. Her translucent teeth and receding gums had caused her dentist great alarm at her last checkup. She was thinking about having a second child but couldn't imagine how she'd cope with a pregnancy in her current state of flat-out exhaustion.

Serena's symptoms at first seemed a clear case of adrenal depletion, but there was a complicating factor: she'd also had digestive problems for years. Fatty foods, in particular, would cause bloating, abdominal pain, and nausea. She found herself gravitating to certain carbs. She often munched on potato chips, Corn Thins, and rice crackers as snacks, and she relied on rice, potatoes, sweet potatoes, and carrots as accompaniments to her meals. She rarely ate breakfast, but when she did she'd opt for "healthy" gluten-free cereals or rice crackers with toppings.

What the Testing Showed

Serena's blood tests showed lowered cortisol and DHEA levels, as I expected, and her poor digestion and potential longer-term malabsorption issues were the result of her low levels of iron and vitamin B_{12}, even though she regularly ate red meat. She also had low levels of homocysteine, zinc, and blood proteins.

Serena's Protocol

I realized that if Serena's adrenal function were to improve, first I had to fix her nutrient stores and improve her digestive power. Her initial treatment plan included an intravenous iron infusion over two visits; monthly vitamin B_{12} injections for three months; zinc, trace elements, multi-B, DHA, and NAC supplements; and Epsom salts foot baths before bed to help her sleep. For digestion, I initially added a fat-digesting enzyme called Lypazyme with each meal.

It took about three months, but these changes made a huge difference in Serena's digestive symptoms and in her energy, allowing her to tolerate more fat and animal proteins. Cutting down on carbs was a struggle, but she was very proud of herself when she was able to do away with the Corn Thins and rice crackers and replace them with "warm salads" loaded with vegetables and a small warm protein, such as fish or tempeh, mixed in. She even discovered mung bean pasta! Serena soon became pregnant, successfully delivered her second child, and is back to being her best at work.

CHAPTER 10

The Optimal Exercise Plan

We all know that exercise is good for us, but there's been little research specifically on its impact during the postnatal period. What is clear is that the combination of plenty of activity, correct movement and posture, and gentle exercises and stretches not only will help your postnatal body to recover its strength, but will also give you more energy, improve your sleep, kick-start your libido, and make you feel so much better.

STRIVING FOR BALANCE IN EXERCISE

You don't need intense, heart-pounding cardio exercise, which can actually be harmful when overdone, to be strong and fit. When you're depleted—and even when you've recovered—less really is more.

The "total physiological load," which refers to our overall state of balance, is particularly important when it comes to exercise. Most exercise has a catabolic (tissue-destructive) effect on our body, but we need an anabolic (tissue-building) capacity as well if we want to remain well balanced, happy, and healthy. Ideally the tissue building and breakdown operate like a seesaw, up and down, before returning to the ideal sensible-middle state. But during this postnatal period, when your body is still adjusting and recovering from major changes, too much of the wrong exercise, too early and too intense, can lead to further depletion.

Think of exercise like a balanced bank account in which the ratio between spending (expending energy/exercising) and saving (rest/recuperation) is constantly changing. Unfortunately, some of us spend without saving, and without regular deposits we can go broke. Being able to move from expending energy to rest and recuperation affects our ability not only to exercise injury-free and enjoy it but also to tone up, get stronger, and shed excess pregnancy weight in due time.

All our body's systems—hormonal, digestive, circulatory, detoxification—interact with one another constantly. And your body doesn't easily distinguish between the physical and biochemical stress from surgery (like a C-section), lack of sleep, or a sore back and the emotional stress from relationship challenges, whether with a partner or a cranky boss. It's all just stress to your body! You might find it harder to recover from an injury, have a lot of aches and pains, or suffer from mood swings and other ailments if you spend too much time in a catabolic state. If so, the last thing you should say is, "I'm so unfit and really should exercise more." The *opposite* is actually true!

HOW AND WHEN TO START EXERCISING AFTER PREGNANCY

The American Congress of Obstetricians and Gynecologists recommends a number of postnatal types of exercise and movement. These gentle low-impact exercises avoid explosive/quick acceleration movements with sudden directional changes—so there's a lower risk of injury, particularly to joints and ligaments. They also tend to improve your circulation, cardiovascular health, and joint range of motion. The recommended exercises include the following:

- Brisk walking
- Swimming
- Aqua aerobics
- Yoga
- Cycling
- Pilates
- Low-impact aerobic workouts
- Light weight training

Physical Readiness

Usually, after the six-week postnatal mark, when your postbaby body is getting back to normal, it is recommended that you get at least 150 minutes of moderate-intensity aerobic activity every week. For physical readiness, depending on your overall health status and your recovery post labor, I offer a few guidelines.

If you had a healthy pregnancy and a normal vaginal delivery, you should be able to start walking again soon after the baby is born. Keep your walking routine slow and gradual. For example, begin with a fifteen-minute walk and then build up to longer walks or more frequent activity. During the first week after delivery, it's important that you closely monitor yourself for vaginal bleeding; unusual fatigue, pain, or swelling of any sort; and shortness of breath. If these symptoms occur, seek medical advice promptly. If in doubt, always reach out to a medical provider to discuss your activities.

If you had a C-section or other complications, ask your doctor when it's safe to begin exercising again. *Medical clearance should precede any exercise regimen.*

When you first start exercising after childbirth, try simple postnatal exercises like pelvic tilts and gentle core exercises, as described on page 204. These will help strengthen the pelvic floor and your major muscle groups, including the abdominal and back muscles. From here, you can gradually build up to other low-impact activities, like swimming, yoga, or Pilates.

Monitor your fatigue levels, as you'll need to adjust your exercise intensity, duration, or frequency when you're very tired. And be patient with fitness progress. Many women, including athletes, do not return to prepregnancy fitness levels for up to two years, and that's okay.

Emotional Readiness

Everyone is different, so you'll need to become attuned to your own level of emotional readiness before returning to exercise. If you are finding that getting motivated, getting prepared, or recovering from exercise is causing a deep sense of unease and stress, then I suspect you may not be ready.

Ilse, the wonderful movement therapist who works in my clinic, told me that prior to the birth of her baby, she played in a competitive rugby union (she was *buff*!), competed as a snowboarder, was a windsurfing instructor, and knew nearly all of her friends through sports. Yet once her daughter was born, she just wasn't that interested in exercise.

"A return to sports was the last thing on my mind," she told me. "Sleep and sanity were ranked on the top of my list for a very long time, and in all honesty, they still are. If it wasn't for my friend Kim, who desperately needed some yoga students, it might have taken me much longer before doing formal exercise. Inde, my daughter, was four at that stage. Once I became a mum, gentle forms of movement like walking, biking with my girl in a seat, and gentle yoga felt much more nurturing to my soul."

Avoiding Injuries

Besides assessing your readiness for exercise, you should also consider *which* exercise form will get you to your goal—whether it's feeling better physically or mentally, having more energy, improving your strength, toning up, and/or shedding weight—in an injury-free manner.

From an orthopedic perspective, women are more prone to injury than men. This is because female hips are wider, leg and knee alignments (the so-called Q angle) are different, and even the angle of the pelvis (anterior pelvic tilt) is slightly bigger. Add to that a higher incidence of joint laxity, much more so around pregnancy and birth, and women are more prone to different injuries.

A graded approach to exercise can really help you avoid unnecessary injury or pain. The illustration on the following page explains in detail the building blocks of intelligent exercise.

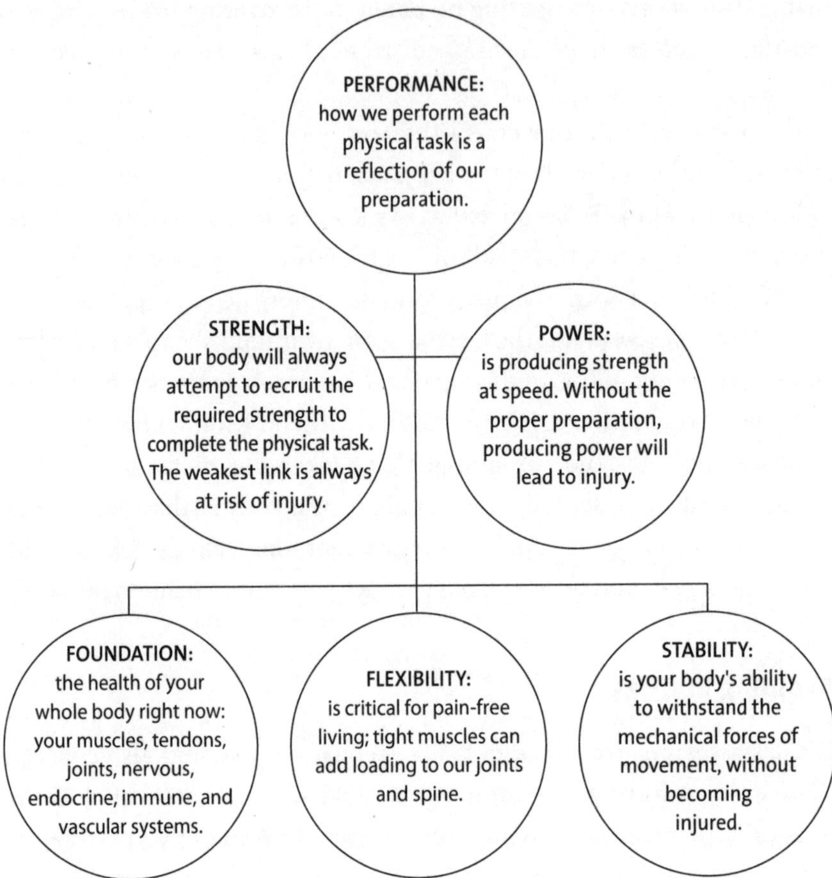

STANDING TALL TO IMPROVE YOUR POSTURE

Posture isn't just about standing and sitting straight. It is also about moving in an ideal way and when you are resting, having a posture that more easily allows bodily processes such as digestion. Correct posture and correct movement can contribute to improved health and well-being. So it's important to work on your posture before you start exercising—and pay attention to it 24/7!

Besides making you look taller and slimmer, good posture helps your

- Mood (it's harder to feel down when you lift your chest)
- Energy levels
- Joints, like those in the neck and shoulders (aligned joints are happy joints)
- Breathing ability, which affects your overall health status
- Quality of movement

Few of us are blessed with naturally good posture, and motherhood is a surefire way of enhancing any postural weaknesses and imbalances you may have. Many moms get in a habit of carrying their little one on one hip (often the same one), while using their one free arm for their daily activities. Carrying a toddler while lugging home a few bags of groceries is guaranteed to leave your neck and back aching. Couple this with limited energy and seated feeding postures, and you might acquire some muscle imbalance.

Muscle imbalances refer to the tendency of different muscles to respond to stress in different ways; some may shorten and tighten while others may lengthen and become prone to weakness. This affects the underlying joints by forcing them out of proper alignment and contributes to pain and dysfunction.

Some exercises can actually worsen posture. Abdominal crunches, for example, can shorten the rectus abdominus muscle, and when this happens, it pulls down the rib cage, leading to an excessive rounding of the spine. Not only can this rounded, slouched posture throw your back out of balance, but it also makes it harder to breathe well. You can test this yourself by sitting tall and taking a few nice, deep breaths; then slouch and try to breathe again. Did you notice how much harder it was to inhale well? There goes your energy! Also, as the neck muscles now need to work harder to help you inhale, they can become excessively tight, leading to pain—and adding another drain on your depleted body.

If you struggle to carry your head in proper alignment—imagine a line running down the side of your body, through your earlobe, the middle of your shoulder, and the hip joint—and no matter what you do, you find that you carry your head farther forward than ideal, please check your breathing. You might be a mouth breather—a common but frequently missed cause of faulty posture.

Ideally, we breathe through our mouths only when we exert, but if this happens during sleep, you might want to get it further assessed, as it is very stressful to the body. Snoring, waking up with a dry mouth, and finding a dribble on your pillow are giveaway signs of mouth breathing. Faulty breathing, however, can show up as a vast array of symptoms, including fatigue, headaches, anxiety, eyestrain, a foggy head, muscle aches and pains, and more. If you know your breathing is not great, follow the food recommendations in the previous chapters to see if breathing through your nose becomes easier, and practice the breathing exercises in chapter 7. If snoring or mouth breathing remains an issue, please see a trained professional. The good news is that there are simple ways to correct muscle imbalances and posture.

What Good Posture Looks Like

In an ideal posture, an imaginary line runs down the side of your body, through the earlobe, the middle of the shoulder, and the hip and knee joints, and falls just before the ankle bone.

Is that how you stand? Even as you read this, quickly check your posture. Are you hunched over when you're feeding the baby or pushing the stroller? Do you slump at your desk? Is your furniture ergonomically supportive?

Many of us are unaware of our posture. It's not until we catch ourselves in the mirror or see a family picture that we notice the way we hold ourselves up. Turning unawareness into an aware body sensation will lead to the biggest changes in your posture. Don't underestimate incidental movement like sitting, standing, carrying your baby, or lifting. These are all opportunities to strengthen good posture and move well. Even better, these incidental "exercises" can be done anytime, anywhere. No tools needed. Just awareness!

How to Get Great Posture

The first thing to do is to become aware of your posture. Feel for a moment what is normal for you. Try this sitting as well as standing.

- Go to a wall and stand with your buttocks against it. Place your shoulder blades against the wall, with your feet a few inches away from the wall. Allow your knees to soften as you elongate your neck.
- Close your eyes and sense what this posture *feels* like. Closing your eyes helps you become attuned to your body's internal navigation system, called proprioception. This ability enables us to know where our limbs are in space without having to look. It is important in all everyday movements but especially so in more complicated movements where precise coordination is essential, like lifting a moving toddler out of a car seat for the fourth time that day! Take note of your head, your chest, your shoulders, and so on. Note if your weight is equally distributed. How about your spinal arches? Is there a difference between the left side and the right side of your lower back? Test this by placing your left hand between the wall and the left side of your spine and then repeat on the right side. Keep your buttocks and back placement steady but natural.
- An *ideal* alignment of the lower back and pelvis is just one hand width of space, measured at your knuckles, between your lower back and the wall. Anything more will add extra loading on your back and body.
- If there is an imbalance, you want to correct this though stretching and strengthening *prior* to loading up your spine. It is best to avoid impactful exercises (jumping, running, weight lifting, etc.).
- If you feel comfortable (and your floor space is clear of toys and obstacles), take a small step forward, away from the wall, with your eyes closed. Do this only if you feel safe. Try to maintain, to

the best of your ability, your nice, tall posture, and *sense* this new feeling. You can visualize an image or think of a word that feels connected to this new posture.

STRETCHING

Stretching feels great and is a terrific way to increase your bodily awareness and sense any areas that might need some TLC before they become problematic. Be aware that in the first four weeks after your baby is born, higher levels of relaxin, the hormone that helps loosen up the pelvis for birth, will still be in your system. So stretching is *not* recommended during this time.

The Benefits of Stretching

- It reduces the risk of injury by reducing muscle imbalances.
- It restores good posture.
- It improves the ability to perform daily tasks like reaching behind your backseat for lost toys.
- It improves the body's ability to pump fluids and detoxify effectively.
- It helps us breathe better, leaving us more energized.

How to Maximize Your Stretching

- Stretch when your body is warm, not cold, to avoid overstretching and injuring a muscle.
- Wear loose, nonrestrictive clothing.
- If a muscle does not feel tight, *do not stretch it.* We all have different levels of flexibility, and it's easy to overstretch and injure joints and their surrounding structures.
- Stay well hydrated by drinking high-quality filtered water.
- Stretch from the top down. If limited with time, do your neck and shoulder stretches before your leg stretches.

- Close your eyes in order to better tune in to any areas of tightness. Not only will you be able to focus your senses inward; it will promote relaxation of your body and mind.
- To facilitate this inward process and relaxation, aim to relax your jaw, mouth, and facial muscles.
- Breathe through the nose. This not only filters and warms the air we inhale; it helps the nervous system to relax (moving from a fight/flight or freeze state into a repair and rest state).
- For an evening stretch routine that addresses common tight muscles from carrying the baby on one hip or seated breastfeeding, go to page 213.

THE BEST FORMS OF POSTNATAL EXERCISE

In our current fast-paced world, we seem to spend a lot of time in our heads while ignoring our bodies and their many messages. This means our bodies miss not only the cues about knowing *where* they are (such as bumping into things, dragging your feet, tripping, and stepping very heavily, causing undue impact on your ankles, knees, and hips) but also what they need to do—such as take a bath, decline an invitation, or lie down for a rest. The more connected you become to your own body by listening to it, the more able you'll be to restore your depletion and harvest your own potential. Slow-movement practices, like restorative yoga, *qigong*, and balancing work, are great to accelerate bodily awareness. Lap swimming, stretching, dancing, and walking mediation are also great ways to bring us back into the body.

Swimming

The beauty of swimming is that it can be done at any pace that suits you. For many people, swimming is an incredibly enjoyable form of exercise on account of the weightlessness you experience in the water as well as the sensory feedback you get from the sensation of the water on your skin. Water itself is thought to be a very healing environment.

Swimming is a low-impact, gentle form of exercise. It is fantastic for breathing and relatively easy to establish your own rhythmic movement in the water. The backstroke is particularly good for opening up the chest, the breaststroke is more soothing, and freestyle (crawl) is perfect for when you're ready to increase your fitness level. All the strokes build strength and release tension in the back of the body and neck.

Swimming is ideally done in a natural low-toxic environment, such as an ocean or a lake, but that can be impractical. Better to swim laps in a chlorinated pool than not at all!

To help reduce absorption of chlorine through the skin, I recommend that mothers take 2 to 4 g vitamin C orally, 30 to 60 minutes before a swim. Having adequate levels of iodine, fat-soluble nutrients such as vitamins D and E, and ALA (alpha linolenic acid, an antioxidant that helps with cell metabolism) will also be protective. Bentonite clay baths are very useful in helping reduce the chlorine odor that lingers after a swim in a pool.

Walking

Walking is the exercise of choice for many mothers, because it's easy to bring the baby along. Many physiotherapists will recommend walking because it is low impact and gentle on the joints. One stroller-walking study noted that new moms valued the ability to get out of the house (26 percent) while having interaction with other mothers (51 percent), and the majority (93 percent) felt it had the potential to increase physical and mental well-being. Which it does! The mothers in the stroller-walking group improved their fitness levels and reduced their level of depressive symptoms significantly more than the control group.

Look for a Mommy & Me walking group in your community, or even start your own. Having the additional support will make you much more likely to get out of the house, move, and feel better. The fresh air will benefit both you and your baby.

As I am a big fan of earthing practices, I recommend walking barefoot whenever possible. In my opinion, nothing beats a barefoot walk in the shallow waves on the beach, breathing in the sea breezes, but if you live in or near a city, invest in a good pair of comfortable shoes and take pleasure in putting them on when going for your daily walk. Try to find a green environment, such as a park, which will feel more uplifting and better for your psychological well-being.

Once your energy levels are returning, you can alternate your walking speeds: start out leisurely, then speed up for a few minutes, then return to a leisurely pace. Try to breathe through your nose and always exercise pain-free. Adding a walk up a small hill or steps can add variation to your walk, but only if you're ready—meaning you have enough energy and no pain.

If you are pain-free, you can add some *small* lunges to your walk by bending your front knee to a 20- or 30-degree angle. Even a few lunges will help your balance and leg strength. To protect your joints, make sure your knee tracks over your second toe and is not falling inward.

If you feel stressed, a walking meditation can do wonders. Slowly move from your thinking head into your sensing, moving body. Aim to see, sense, hear, and smell the world around you through mindful awareness.

Yoga

There are many different forms of yoga, all of which will greatly help your breath awareness and flexibility. However, some yoga styles, such as vinyasa or hot yoga (classes built around a dynamic sequence of poses) will not be suitable when you're depleted. You might want to stick to extremely gentle forms of yoga for quite some time, even years. Don't feel that you have to push or strain yourself. Allow yourself to find a yoga practice that feels right for you.

I've found that many people are resistant to the thought of yoga without even trying it. This is really a shame, as it can be a powerful healing tool. Ilse and I both believe that the more tools people have in their toolbox, the more easily they'll find *something* that will resonate with them that they can turn into helpful new habits.

Giving birth and the transition that follows open every new parent up to new possibilities, as they can't help but look at life differently. This can unlock their potential to become an even more powerful and potent person. The experience of yoga—in which we invite the self inward and, through breathing, reconnect with our bodies in the present moment—is a beautiful gift you can give yourself. So I hope you try it!

Make Your Muscles Stronger

You need a strong upper body to perform the essential daily baby tasks. Lifting the baby umpteen times a day, holding the baby, carrying the baby, and pushing the baby in a stroller means that you are constantly engaging your upper-body muscles. The stronger they are, the easier (and safer) it will be for you. You also need a strong core, which is the foundation of all strength in your body, to support the work of your spine. Your core muscles were sorely taxed during pregnancy and will need some attention to regain their strength.

Free Weights

From a functional perspective, using free weights to tone up and increase your strength far outweighs the use of machine-based fitness found in gyms. When you use your own body, without being locked into a machine, you train your balance, coordination, and integration of your brain and body. This will carry over into your daily life as you find yourself squatting while lifting a heavy laundry basket or picking up a moving toddler in a parking lot. You will be less likely to lose your balance or injure yourself when you've built up some strength.

If weight loss is on your mind, please note that lifting weights is much more effective than running on a treadmill because you are using many muscle groups at once. If done intelligently, using free weights is less stressful to the overall nervous system than is pounding away endlessly on a treadmill. It also builds bone density, fine-tunes your balance, and increases the muscle mass that will speed up your metabolism.

Don't worry about bulking up, because women just don't have the same testosterone levels as men. Do, however, seek out a certified personal trainer to walk you through the proper form for any weight training. It is essential to correct your posture before loading the spine and other joints with any weights. If you are noticing any pain at all, especially in your wrists, back, or neck, do the postnatal exercises on page 201 before you start weight training.

Stability or Swiss balls can be great tools for the same purpose and allow you to do various functional exercises from the convenience of your home.

If you like cardiovascular work, it is best to do it *after* your strength training. This way you are less likely to get injured.

Core Training

Ilse is a physiotherapist, personal trainer, and Pilates instructor, and she's often told me how amazed she is by how many people injure themselves or suffer from back, leg, and arm injuries due to poor core function. It doesn't matter where they're exercising—the gym, at home, outside, even in Pilates or yoga classes—they still get hurt.

There are several reasons for this. First, many people don't know what the core muscles are, how to target them, and what constitutes proper core technique. In addition, if you are struggling with digestive problems (bloating, burping, loose bowels, etc.), your body will likely create space to accommodate these struggling organs, shutting down the core muscles in the process.

The most important deeper core muscles (sometimes referred to as the inner unit) consist of the transverse abdominus (TVA), multifidus, pelvic floor, and diaphragm. This inner unit operates on a different neurological loop from other core muscles, and they have the ability to influence one another. This means you can reduce urinary incontinence by activating the right core muscle!

To better understand this concept, think of the muscles as lights all controlled by one switch. Try the following exercise: Place a couple of fingers between your legs just in front of your rectum. Now draw your belly button toward your spine as though you were sucking your tummy in to get on a pair of tight pants. You should feel your pelvic floor tighten up.

If the TVA (the deepest, most inner layer of all abdominals) is working properly, it will contract before the extremities move, stabilizing the spine and pelvis. If it does not work correctly, it will be unable to support your spine, limbs, pelvis, and pelvic floor! Many consequences come from ignoring this important functional muscle.

Increase Your TVA Awareness

The TVA—Gentle Core Work, exercise 2 on page 205, is the best. You can't overdo this gentle yet effective exercise, which shapes your core in a safe, functional way. You can also add pelvic floor exercises to strengthen the workings of the inner unit. This preparation will pay off as you progress to other forms of exercise. Much like designing a good foundation for your home, if you do this exercise well, you can build anything on top of it.

If, despite proper technique, you struggle to recruit this muscle, seek professional help before commencing more strenuous exercise. You may first need to address other factors that might affect your core, such as digestive complaints, constipation, stress or pain from surgery, or birth trauma.

CORRECTING COMMON POSTNATAL CHALLENGES

There are several common postnatal challenges that require additional care, and fortunately these gentle exercises will help reduce these conditions. As always, avoid pain or discomfort and *seek professional advice if your condition is not improving.* If in doubt, reach out!

Postnatal Incontinence and Kegel Exercises

About 58 percent of those who had a vaginal delivery and 43 percent of those who had a C-section experience some form of pelvic floor dysfunction. Unfortunately, most women also suffer in silence, despite the fact that a weakened pelvic floor isn't just about inconvenience—it can affect activity levels and sexual function. This is very common after deliver, and if you can receive correct information and instruction early, you should be able to fully reestablish the stability of your pelvic floor.

Incontinence refers to lack of voluntary control over urination or defecation. Most new moms suffer from stress incontinence, which occurs when pelvic muscles have been damaged or weakened, causing the bladder to leak during exercise, coughing, sneezing, laughing, or any other body movement that puts pressure on the bladder.

Urinary stress incontinence is very common; American research shows that 34 percent of new moms suffer with it. About 40 percent of women experience significant nerve-related pain that usually resolves within six months. The pelvic floor region is a perfect example of why it's important to ease into exercise and be highly attuned to the changes in your body. Exercises involving repetitive bouncing are associated with the highest incidence of incontinence. If you're worried about accidents, switch from exercises that cause urine loss (jumping, jogging, and running) to low-impact activities, such as walking, cycling, swimming, and weight training.

Know Your Pelvic Floor Muscles

The floor of the pelvis is made up of layers of muscle and other tissues. These layers stretch like a hammock from your pubic bone to your tailbone. Your pelvic floor muscles support your bladder, uterus, and colon; in addition to helping you control your bladder and bowel, they aid sexual function. These muscles are an important part of your deeper core muscles. Besides pregnancy and labor, pelvic floor muscles can be affected by constipation, heavy lifting, weakened abdominal muscles, excess weight, and chronic coughing.

Kegel Exercises

Kegel exercises are one of the best ways to strengthen the pelvic floor and reduce urinary stress incontinence. They can also assist the healing of the perineum by improving circulation.

To be successful at pelvic floor muscle training, you must know how to contract the correct muscles. The key to doing Kegels correctly is to locate them correctly. The easiest way to do this is, while urinating, to stop the urine from flowing by tightening or squeezing your muscles. Those are the muscles to clench and unclench during Kegels. If you find that clenching the muscles minimizes but does not stop the urine flow, you have found the right muscles, but you also know that they are weak—a good indication to practice!

Another way to locate these muscles is during sexual activity. Place your index and middle fingers inside your vagina in a slight V shape. Now squeeze around your fingers; the muscle you tighten is the exact muscle you'll want to contract and relax during the Kegel exercises.

- Sit, stand, or lie down with your legs, thighs, buttocks, and abdominal muscles relaxed. (Initially, lying down might be easier.)
- Take a deep breath, and on the exhale, contract your pelvic floor muscles, drawing them up inside. Think high!
- Hold for ten seconds, then relax for ten seconds. Fully let go.
- Varying the speed of your contractions by tightening and holding for two seconds, then relaxing for two seconds, can be interspersed with the longer ten-second hold. Remember that a few strong contractions are always better than many weaker ones. Do plenty of Kegels during the day.

When you first start this exercise, you might move your pelvis or feel your buttock muscles contract. As you practice, you'll likely become better at isolating the right muscles, keeping the inner-thigh, abdominal, and buttock action separate from your pelvic floor contraction. Each repetition will increase the strength of the muscles. In time, doing your Kegels will become easier. If you still have trouble after doing the exercises in this section (as well as the TVA exercise starting on page 205) because you aren't sure about your ability to contract the right muscles, your symptoms don't change, or you experience pain, ask for help.

Be sure to pay equal attention to both the contraction and the relaxation of the muscle. It's much better to practice Kegels while *exhaling*—you'll be less likely to bear down, adding strain on your pelvic floor. Kegel exercises alternated with gentle abdominal exercise, like Horse

Stance (see exercise 5 on page 206), will speed up the healing process and pelvic floor recovery.

Relieving Postnatal Pain with Gentle Exercise

There are certain kinds of pain that are common during and after pregnancy. If you have pain that does not subside, worsens, is severe, or keeps you up at night, you must seek professional medical advice, as it is highly unlikely that the pain will go away on its own!

Lower Back Pain

Numerous studies have shown that 50 to 90 percent of pregnant women experience some type of back pain due, not surprisingly, to the extra load on your spine coupled with the hormones that loosen your ligaments.

It's important to have good stability, flexibility, and posture prior to doing strength exercises, which will allow you to recover from low back pain much faster. Swimming, walking, breathing, and relaxing exercises are all fantastic choices to minimize or eliminate lower back pain, as are water-based exercise programs. Gentle stretches starting a month or so after birth can also be helpful. Avoid abdominal crunches from the floor, leg-lowering exercises (which you might do in a Pilates class or at the gym), and any other exercise that taxes your back.

Hand and Wrist Pain

Hand pain, primarily from carpal tunnel syndrome (CTS), is the second-most-frequent musculoskeletal symptom of pregnancy. Usually, it causes pain and numbness on both sides of the hand, especially in the thumbs. Pregnancy-related CTS is often caused by excess fluid, so water activities, like swimming and hydrotherapy, may reduce symptoms.

CTS can continue once your pregnancy is over, though. Carrying and lifting your baby countless times during the day can stress a still-recovering body. Repetitive wrist movements and exercises that cause strain on the wrist joints can further aggravate your pain, so try to avoid them.

Exercising in water is very helpful in the postnatal period, as the buoyancy will help to unload your joints while the resistance of the water will safely strengthen your body.

Gentle stretching of the forearm, shoulders, and neck and maintaining an optimum posture are both helpful. You may need to modify your lifting, too. Carry your baby close to your body (slings are great for this) while maintaining good leg strength. Remember to bend your knees and lift from your legs instead of from your arms and back. Try modifying your breastfeeding posture by lying down rather than sitting so that your hands, wrists, and arms can rest.

Diastasis Recti—Separation of the Abdominal Muscles

Separation (or diastasis) of the rectus abdominus muscle (located in the midline of the belly) is another common issue during pregnancy. Although a significant improvement without the need for intervention will usually occur on its own, separation may continue in some women. If you notice bulging in the midline of the abdominal wall during exercises or as you go to sit up in bed, you might have some level of abdominal widening. You can get a sense of the extent of it by feeling with your fingers for a gap as you lie down with your knees flexed while raising your head toward your knees. If you do notice a widening, have it assessed by your midwife or physician.

If you have a diastasis wider than three fingers, take special care to build up your abdominal muscles more slowly and to avoid stressing the area. Don't do any abdominal crunches, in which you lift your entire upper back off the floor. Also avoid heavy lifting and other strenuous exercise. Instead, do Kegel exercises every day as well as exercises 1, 2, 3, and 5, starting on page 204. Once you have done these for six to eight weeks, you can add these modified curl-ups:

- Place your hands on either side of the diastasis recti and maintain some gentle pressure, moving toward the midline.
- Take a nice deep breath in, then draw your belly button toward your spine on your exhale, while you slowly and gently lift your

head and shoulders off the floor—just a little! Keep your waist on the floor at all times. To protect your neck, keep your tongue on the roof of your mouth. Your trunk should always remain connected to the floor. The curling-up action is supported by the drawing in and up motion of your belly button to your spine. Move up only on the exhale.

- To exercise all parts of the abdominal muscles, the curl-ups are done in both a straight way and a diagonal manner. During diagonal curl-ups, move exactly as above, then turn your shoulder a little toward your opposite knee. Still maintain hand contact and lift only the head and shoulders.

Exercising after a C-Section

Make sure your physician says it's okay before starting any exercise. Once you are given permission, start with gentle pelvic floor exercises and stabilizing exercises 1, 2, 3, and 5 starting on page 204. You can add exercise 6 (see page 207), very gently, after six to eight weeks, making sure to avoid excess stretching of the surgical site. With all forms of exercise, continue to breathe throughout the exercise. This will reduce any extra strain on the abdomen and pelvic floor.

As long as your scar has healed well, which will be assessed during your postsurgery and postnatal checkups, it can be a good idea to do water-based work. Regular walking is great, too, as it will stimulate spinal movement, circulation, and deeper breathing.

Also, when your physician gives you the go-ahead, start to massage your scar a few minutes every day. You can use rose hip oil, which improves surgical scars and prevents the formation of keloids (excess tissue) after surgical procedures, or coconut oil.

Varicose Veins

Varicose veins are probably the last thing you want to think about right now, yet appropriate exercise can minimize them.

While the quality of your veins (and all tissue) is greatly influenced by the quality of your overall health, as your core and pelvic floor weaken during pregnancy, the abdominal organs can drop down (called visceral ptosis). This extra load can compromise blood flow, predisposing you to varicose veins.

Stay away from machine-based exercises, such as leg presses and Spinning, as they pump blood up to the pelvis while the torso moves very little. Non-machine-based pelvic floor and stabilizing exercises are a better choice, as are whole-body exercises like yoga and stretching.

The Postnatal Exercise Program

When you first start exercising after childbirth, try simple postnatal exercises that help strengthen major muscle groups, including your abdominal and back muscles. Use your own body as resistance before you add any weights.

These exercises progress from easy to moderate. If in doubt, stick to exercises 1 to 6, which follow, and the evening TLC stretching routine (see page 213). Gradually work your way through the other corrective exercises. *Only progress with exercises if you can do so pain-free.* It's much more helpful to work out in good form, with less weight, than to do more challenging exercises in poor form. You will not do your body any favors by overtaxing it.

1. *Pelvic Tilt—Gentle Core Work*

Benefits: This exercise reconnects your lower back to your pelvis and strengthens your abdominals in a gentle way.

- Lie on your back on the floor with your knees bent.
- Feel the small gap between your back and the floor.
- As you exhale, flatten your lower spine against the floor by drawing your belly button to your spine. This should feel like a slight upward lift.
- Release as you inhale again.
- Repeat five times and work up to ten to twenty repetitions per session.

2. *TVA—Gentle Core Work*

Benefits: This exercise is a great way to learn how to use your deep core muscles. It activates the TVA, the muscle that shapes your belly, and provides important support to your spine, internal organs, and pelvic floor muscles. Most people find that a gentle activation of the TVA works best. They are less like to tighten the abdominals excessively or hold their breath.

- Kneel on the floor with your shoulders and hips directly above your hands and knees. Take a slow, even breath in.
- Exhale and draw your belly button toward your spine and upward—like a lifting motion.
- On the out breath, pull up and in and then continue to breathe as normal.
- Keep the lower spine in a neutral position, remaining still.
- Repeat ten times, each time holding for ten seconds.

3. *Heel Slides—Gentle Core Work*

Benefits: Heel slides are a great integration exercise for the lower abdominals and lower extremities.

- Lie down with your back on the floor, shoes off.
- Have your hips and knees flexed (relatively close to the buttocks).
- Place your spine in a neutral position, leaving a hand width of space at the level of your knuckles.
- Leave your hand in the hollow of your back, close your eyes, and take a deep diaphragmatic breath.
- Slowly exhale and draw your belly button in toward your spine.
- After exhalation slowly slide your left leg out away from the start position.
- If the pressure on your hand begins to increase or decrease, *stop* the movement and slide your leg back to the beginning position.
- Practice both sides, in good form only.

Note: Make a note of the distance of your outstretched leg. As you learn how to control your core muscles, you will slowly be able to move your leg farther away. I can't stress enough the importance of practicing with good form! It is better to do three proper heel slides on each side than twenty poor ones.

4. *Cat Camel—Spinal Movement*

Benefits: The gentle arching and rounding of the spine increases spinal awareness, spinal movement, and spinal health while also aiding in relaxation. Start gently and *move only in pain-free range.*

- Get down on all fours, with your wrists and knees directly under your shoulders and hips, respectively. If this position causes wrist pain, place your fists on the floor instead.
- As you inhale, gently look up and arch your spine.
- As you exhale, round your spine, tucking your tailbone, pushing your shoulders away from the floor, and allowing the neck to fully relax.
- After a few rounds, for increased body awareness and relaxation, close your eyes.
- As your body warms up, increase the depth of your breath, keeping your mouth and jaw relaxed.
- Repeat until your movement feels fluid and free. Slow is better.

5. *Horse Stance—Multifidus—Back Training*

Benefits: This exercise trains the small muscles around your spine, important for pain-free lifting, bending, and rotating.

- While on all fours, place your wrists and knees directly under your shoulders and hips, respectively, with your fingers facing forward.
- Place a dowel rod along your spine and hold in perfect alignment.
- The space between your lower back and the rod should be about the thickness of your hand.
- Activate your deep core muscle (TVA) by drawing the belly button in, toward your spine.

- Lift one hand off the floor just enough to slide an envelope between your hand and the floor.
- Lift your opposite knee the same way.
- Remain as stable as you can. Hold for ten seconds, then release and switch sides.
- Do as many repetitions as you can, in good form only.

6. *Yogi Bridge—Spinal Awareness*

Benefits: This gentle exercise aids proprioception. It is a great for relaxation and can reduce back and pelvic-related pain.

- Lie on your back with your hips and knees bent. Your heels are relatively close to the buttocks.
- Keep your legs parallel to each other, and your palms facing up.
- With closed eyes, gently lengthen your tailbone by drawing your belly button to your spine.
- Aim to lift one vertebra at a time off the floor, like you are peeling your spine from the floor.
- Slow is better—aim to feel for fluid movement.
- Roll back down in a similar manner, dropping one segment at a time back onto the floor.
- Repeat until your motion is fluid and well controlled.
- Do not hold your breath.
- If you experience any pain, squeeze your buttock muscles or contract your pelvic floor.

7. *Bridge—Gentle Glute Strength*

Benefits: This exercise helps with back, pelvic, hip, and knee pain while toning up the buttocks.

- Lying on your back with your hips and knees bent (heels are relatively close to the buttocks).
- Legs are shoulder-width apart, palms facing up.
- Gently press your hips up while bearing your weight through your heels.

- Hold for ten seconds, then lower.
- Repeat until muscle fatigue.
- If you feel this in your lower back, squeeze your buttock muscles or lower your hips slightly.

8. *Bridge + Resistance Band—Gentle Glute Strength*

Benefits: This exercise helps with back, pelvic, hip, and knee pain while toning up the buttocks and strengthening the pelvic floor.

- Follow the first 2 steps in exercise 7, adding an elastic resistance band.
- Place the band around your thighs, just above your knees, nice and snug.
- Place your hips and knees shoulder-width apart—this will create tension on the band, felt as resistance.
- Follow the last 4 steps of exercise 7 while maintaining tension on the band at all times.

Progression: You can place your baby on your hip or lower tummy while doing this exercise. *Make sure to hold on to the little one so you are both safe!*

9. *Single Leg Bridge—Advanced Glute Strength*

Benefits: This exercise helps with back, hip, and leg strength and is great for toning up safely.

- Lie on your back with your hips and knees bent (heels are relatively close to the buttocks).
- Legs are shoulder-width apart, palms are facing up.
- Gently press your hips up while bearing your weight through your heels.
- Keep your hips level, then lift one leg off the floor.
- Maintain balanced hips to the best of your ability and continue to breathe.
- Hold for ten seconds, then switch legs.
- Continue until muscle fatigue.

Note: If you experience lower-back discomfort, you might want to first work on strengthening your core glutes by doing an easier version of the bridge (try exercise 7 or 8 on pages 207–208). Alternatively, lie on your back, bring both knees to your chest, and hug them for a while to release some back muscle tension. Continue only if you can do so pain-free.

10. *Shoulder Blade Squeeze—Shoulders, Posture*

Benefits: This exercise helps prevent tense shoulders and upper back while cultivating posture awareness.

- Stand with your feet hip-width apart, or sit nice and tall—chest lifted and neck elongated.
- Squeeze your shoulder blades down and toward each other, then release.
- Repeat ten to twenty times.

11. *Alternating Superman on the Floor or on a Swiss Ball—Shoulder and Arm Strength, Posture*

Benefits: This exercise is a great way to improve your posture and prevent or correct posture-related pains (such as neck and shoulder discomfort and headaches caused by a forward head posture).

- Lie on your stomach on the floor or on a ball.
- Keep your head and neck elongated as you look down—place the tongue on the roof of your mouth.
- Keep your arm at a 45-degree angle from your spine with your thumb up.
- Keep your shoulders away from your ears.
- Start with lifting one arm in the above position. Keep your feet on the floor soft as you aim to balance to the best of your abilities.
- Continue to breathe.
- Practice ten times for a ten-second hold each. This will improve postural endurance.

Progression: If you can perform ten single arm lifts for ten seconds, pain-free and in good form (elongated neck, thumb up, and shoulders away from the ears), progress to the following exercise:

- Begin with the same starting position as above.
- Lift the opposite arm and leg *at the same time.* Hold for ten seconds while maintaining good form and continuing to breathe.
- Repeat five times and work up to ten repetitions per session.

12. *Standing Low Row—Shoulder and Arm Strength, Posture*

Benefits: This exercise strengthens your upper arm and shoulder blade region, helping you lift with more ease.

- Stand and hold a weight in your right hand.
- Place your left foot on top of a chair.
- Lean your torso forward so that it is close to your left foot, and rest your left forearm on your thigh to support your back.
- Allow the weight in your right hand to hang down toward the floor.
- Pull your right elbow back along your right side, palm facing toward your torso.
- Aim to use the muscles between your shoulder blades, while keeping your right shoulder low.
- The action is much like starting up a lawn mower (just more gentle—and a lot more quiet!).
- Perform ten repetitions in good form, then switch legs and arms.

13. *Single Leg Biceps—Shoulders, Balance*

Benefits: This exercise strengthens your upper arms and improves your lifting ability while heightening brain/body awareness and lessening injuries.

- Stand nice and tall, chest lifted and neck elongated.
- Balance on your left leg, bringing your right leg in front of you at a 90-degree angle from your hip.
- Maintain softness in your left knee, while your left kneecap faces straight forward.

- Aim to keep your right hip level with the left.
- With dumbbells in both hands, palms up, alternate bringing your hand to your shoulder (left and right separate). Start light, with one- or two-pound weights, and build up only if you can do so pain-free and in good form.
- Do ten repetitions, then switch legs.
- Repeat until muscle fatigue.

Progression: You may gradually increase the weight of the dumbbells, but only if you can do so pain-free and in good form.

14. *Box Step-Up—Leg Strength*

Benefits: This exercise strengthens the muscles around your hips and tones your legs.

- Imagine a line going from your kneecap to over your second toe. Maintain this alignment at all times.
- Maintain good upright posture at all times.
- Keep your hip bones level; do not allow your hips to shift sideways as you step up onto either a stool, a curb, or stairs.
- Alternate legs, equally stepping up with the left and right leg.
- Repeat until muscle fatigue, keeping in mind that your form is more important than your number of repetitions.

Progression: You can increase the step height or do step-ups while holding more weight (such as your baby or a dumbbell). Use steps or curbs to add step-ups to your walking routine. Because your hip joints loosened to facilitate the birth of your baby, they can remain unstable for a little while, so do this progression only when your body strength has improved and there is no pain.

15. *Front Squat—Whole-Body Strength*

Benefits: This exercise helps with everyday activities like lifting your baby or bags of groceries, as it strengthens your lower and upper back.

- Stand tall with your chest lifted. Look forward. Hold a light weight close to your chest.
- Prior to lowering into the squat, draw your belly button toward your spine.
- As you lower yourself by bending your knees, much like a sitting-down motion, make sure to not drop your knee inward.
- Keep your weight equally on both feet, with your feet pointed outward slightly.
- Release air through pursed lips.
- Only lower in a pain-free range.

If you have trouble keeping your heels on the floor or bearing your weight on your left and right sides equally, err on the side of caution. Stretch your leg muscles first until any imbalances are corrected.

16. *Sumo Squat—Whole-Body Strength*

Benefits: This exercise helps with back, pelvic, hip, and knee pain caused by hip-joint instability.

- Stand with your feet wider than hip-width apart.
- Gently bring your belly button toward your spine.
- Focus on using your thighs and buttocks as you slowly lower, bend your knees, and sit back into a squat.
- Keep your chest lifted to the sky and your shoulder blades close together.
- Ideally, your knees track over your second toes. As you come out of the movement, press through your heels and slowly exhale through pursed lips.
- Repeat until muscle fatigue. Remember, form is more important than repetitions.
- Give yourself at least one to two rest days in between strength routines.

POSTNATAL STRENGTH EXERCISES TO AVOID

Avoid these exercises:

Abdominal crunches. They contribute to rounding of the spine, postural-related pain, and suboptimal breathing. (There goes your energy!)

Planks. They are not that functional, and most people are unable to keep good form, which leads to straining.

Leg raises. They are very challenging to do correctly, and doing them incorrectly can contribute to muscle imbalances and pain.

Dips. They are not worth the high injury risk.

Overhead lifts with a suboptimal posture.

If you have low back pain, hip, knee, or leg pain, possibly caused by pelvic/sacroiliac joint instability, avoid the following exercises until you are pain-free:

- Lunges in any direction
- High step-ups and step-downs
- Elliptical trainers
- Stairmasters
- Cycling with the seat too high
- Running
- Pilates exercises in which the legs are farther away from the torso and the core muscles are unable to stabilize your spine and pelvic region

Evening TLC Stretch Routine

My stretch routine is a great way to counteract the muscular imbalances that many moms experience as a result of their daily routines: carrying little ones on one hip, seated feeding, and trying to manage their depletion.

This routine will also help you unwind. Be gentle; stretches should aid relaxation. To more easily soften into your stretches, make sure you are well hydrated and comfortable (wearing warm, loose-fitting clothing, etc.). Aim to bring your awareness inward—I can't overemphasize the benefits of doing this practice.

To get the most out of these stretches, follow these guidelines: Close your eyes and soften your jaw and mouth. (Closing our eyes signals to our bodies that we're relaxed.) If your mind races, wonders, or is agitated, focus on your breath or repeat a positive mantra. Choose any thought that feels good. Soothing music can help, too. If you feel tight around your neck, you'll want to include exercises 1, 2, and 3. If your goal is to unwind after a busy day and give yourself some much-needed TLC, you can go straight to exercise 4. Follow the exercises in the order given here, and make note of your favorite ones, knowing that you can come back to the practice at any time.

1. *Head Muscles*

- Sit or stand comfortably, aware of your posture—straight and tall.
- Place your nondominant hand on your chin and your dominant hand just under your skull, at the top of your neck, with your elbow facing up to the sky.
- Slowly inhale while gently lengthening the upper spine with your dominant hand. As you inhale, your chin might want to come forward. Resist this gently with your nondominant hand.
- Hold for three to five deep breaths.

2. *Neck*

- Sit or stand comfortably, aware of your posture—straight and tall.
- Reach one arm as far down between your shoulder blades as possible.
- Look as far as you comfortably can to the opposite side.
- Take in a deep breath and hold it for five seconds.
- As you exhale, look downward as far as you can comfortably toward your shoulder.
- Repeat on the other side.

3. *Upper Shoulders*

- Sit or stand comfortably straight and tall with your back against a wall.
- With your nose straight forward, drop your right ear to your right shoulder, and relax your neck into the stretch you'll feel on the lengthened, left side of your neck. If there is any neck discomfort, bring your chin slightly closer to your chest, aiming to remain tall. Gently soften your breath, your jaw, and your mouth.
- Hold the stretch for twenty to thirty seconds.
- Repeat on the other side.

4. *Long-Lie Chest Opener*

- Lie on a foam roller, yoga bolster, or rolled-up blanket with your palms facing up. Your head, upper spine, and tailbone are touching the bolster.
- Breathe in from the belly, allowing your lower ribs to expand sideways.
- Place one hand on your belly to feel it rise. Then place this hand, palm facing up, next to your torso again.
- Your neck and shoulders are resting and soft, and your jaw is relaxed.
- Close your eyes and allow your body to soften using your breath, while slowly opening your chest.
- Remain in this position for as long as you feel comfortable.

5. *Upper-Body Rotation*

- Lie on your side with a rolled-up towel or small firm pillow under your head.
- With your knees together, bring them in front so your thighs are bent at a 90-degree angle from the hip. Keep your feet together.
- Bring both hands together as you extend your arms out from your shoulders.

- On an inhale, slide your top hand with very little effort over the bottom one toward your shoulder.
- As your hand moves toward the shoulder, begin to twist your spine and exhale. Gently bring your top arm and shoulder to the floor while keeping your hips, knees, and lower body still.
- You can slowly turn your head or gaze up at the sky or ceiling.
- Rest here for three breaths, then inhale to rotate back.
- Perform as many repetitions as you need to encourage a gentle lowering of the shoulder to the floor.
- Repeat on the other side.

6. *Trunk and Back Stretch*

- Kneel on all fours, hips above knees, and place one hand in front of the other hand.
- Reach forward and away from your body in a diagonal pattern. Continue to reach forward and across, while your hips stay still, until you feel a stretch at the side of your torso. If there is any discomfort in the top of your shoulder, gently pull back so you are pain-free.
- Allow your head and neck to soften, and hold for three to five breaths.
- Repeat on the other side.

7. *Cross-Legged Side Bend*

- Sit on the floor with your legs comfortably crossed.
- Place your left hand beside your left hip. Inhale as you reach up with your right arm and extend it over your right ear, palm facing the floor.
- Exhale and reach to the left, feeling the stretch on your right side. Continue to lift toward the sky even as you side bend.
- Hold for three to five breaths.
- Repeat on the other side.

8. *Groin and Hamstring Opener*

- Sit with your legs apart, right knee bent, with your right heel at your pubic bone.
- Place your left arm on your left leg, elbow against your knee, palm facing up.
- Reach your right arm overhead toward your left foot.
- Inhale as you reach up. Exhale as you lengthen through your arm and torso.
- Hold for three to five deep breaths.
- Repeat on the other side.

9. *Kneeling Back Stretch*

- Kneel down and sit on your heels.
- Keep your knees about hip-width apart, or wider if you experience any groin pain.
- Place your hands on your thighs.
- Slide your hands down your thighs onto the floor in front of you, supporting your weight as your body moves down toward the floor. If you are able to, you can rest your forehead on the floor.
- Once in this position, place both arms next to your torso, palms facing the ceiling.
- Allow your shoulders and neck to relax to the best of your abilities.
- Breathe slowly and deeply, allowing your back to relax, and adjust your hips as needed.
- Hold for three to five breaths or longer.

PART IV

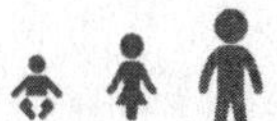

Recovering Your Life

CHAPTER 11

Recovering and Rebuilding Emotional Well-Being

Becoming a mother is one of those life events that changes you irrevocably. For all the love and the joy that comes with having a baby, it can also be fraught with the potential for deeply pervasive negative emotions and thoughts. In addition to your happiness and delight in your newborn, there can be equally intense overwhelming feelings of vulnerability, sadness, isolation, anxiety, and depression. These feelings can be even harder to manage for new moms who have been longing for a child for quite some time—why, they wonder, are they feeling so bad when they finally have the one thing they wanted so much?

Compound these feelings with the physical effects of postnatal depletion, especially sleep deprivation, and you can find yourself in a dark place you never expected.

I hope it will instantly make you feel better when I say that what you are feeling might be tough, but it is totally *normal* and has been experienced by millions upon millions of other mothers, too—even if they kept this roller coaster of despair and worries to themselves.

What I've found the most helpful with my patients is to tackle these emotional issues at the same time we're tackling the physical issues you read about in part 2. Sometimes, but not always, when physical depletion is addressed, many of the overwhelming feelings diminish, too, and very quickly. These patients tell me it was as if they'd been walking through a thick fog that suddenly dissipated—and they were thrilled to be *themselves* again.

But for most patients, physical and emotional issues need to be tackled simultaneously. I've found that a three-pronged approach helps. The first step is to acknowledge the emotional journey you're on and to commit to sharing these feelings with your partner, trusted friends (especially moms who've already gone through similar scenarios), or a professional. The second step aims to reduce negative feelings by putting yourself into the "flow state," a mind-set that will help you better tackle the day-to-day stresses and demands of being a new mom and lead you to happiness. The third step is practicing self-love, which is such an important concept that it deserves, and gets, its own chapter (see chapter 12).

CONFRONTING THE EMOTIONAL JOURNEY OF MOTHERHOOD

Although motherhood is an amazingly rich and satisfying experience like no other, it will always send you off on a twisting, turning road where you'll encounter bumps that you can't foresee. This is due to the physical changes that took place in your brain when you were pregnant, an overnight change in your relationship with your partner, social expectations that you can "do it all," hypervigilance in worrying about infant caretaking (especially if your baby is fussy), sleep deprivation, hormonal shifts, physical depletion, and social isolation.

Now, whom can you turn to for help? Your already overwhelmed partner, endlessly critical mother-in-law, demanding colleagues at the workplace, or a well-meaning yet ineffectual health-care system that finds it easier to prescribe pharmaceuticals you don't need than to sit down and ask you how you're really feeling? No wonder you feel so bad!

But if my patients can improve and recover, and they do, so can you. No matter how bad you are feeling, I have no doubt that you *can* and *will* improve your health—you will recover your vitality and positive state of mind, and you will feel *better* than ever.

All that I'm asking you to do now is be motivated. Believe that you can feel good in your body and in your life again. This is the crucial first step in keeping you off the slippery slope that takes you from mild postnatal issues to severe postnatal depletion.

Ask for Help!

The last thing I want you to feel is alone. You have just become a vital member of the sisterhood of mothers, and you are *not* alone. Our Western society might not have evolved to provide emotional and physical support to all new moms, but there are countless resources for you once you start looking for them. The simple act of sharing your feelings, doubts, and insecurities about your enormous new role will hopefully be a big part of you recovering your emotional stability. This does require sharing some of your vulnerabilities, but there is liberation and support in this.

I do, however, think it is important to be selective about what you share and with whom you decide to connect. The first place to look for connection is in your postnatal support groups—other mothers and/or couples whom you connected or felt an affinity with. Check in with them and see how they're doing. Find out what's working for them or what they're struggling with—and you will likely get honest and helpful answers when you share your own ups and downs. Many moms, as I'm sure you know, try to put on a brave face lest they feel ashamed that they don't have the "perfect" baby and postnatal life they dreamed of, and they are desperately relieved when they can open up to a sympathetic ear.

Also check out what support groups for mothers are in your area—there might be mommy–baby yoga classes, for example, walking mothers' groups, cooking groups, or singing groups. Community centers can often be a great resource for information and often host many events or groups at a low cost. Child-care groups and centers as well as preschools are a great source of contacts and people to connect with, once you negotiate the sometimes palpable competitive energy. If it isn't working with someone or if you feel judged or belittled, be nice but move on. Start to build relationships within the groups and with other parents.

A common theme that I hear from mothers is the loss of connection with their old friends (who may or may not have kids). It is so important to try to maintain these connections in whatever form you can, because these are the people who often know you best. Old friends, especially those who've known you a long time, are priceless, and it is so worthwhile to stay in touch no matter how infrequently you may actually catch up.

If you feel your life has been derailed and you are struggling, it can be hard to open up to your old friends, who you may feel see you in a totally different light. You're going to have to feel comfortable explaining to them that things have changed for you. I often hear beautiful stories of how therapeutic it can be when a struggling mother and her old friends do get together, especially when sharing the challenges, disappointments, expectations, and realities. Not only do mothers feel acknowledged during such get-togethers, but the feedback from their friends is often invaluable, with insights and solutions that may have been invisible to the mothers.

If your old friends live near you, plan ahead and try to have special get-togethers even if they're only every few months—anything from a girls' night out to having a massage/facial/pedicure date, going for a walk, or sharing a meal. What you do can be a lot of fun, but the real value lies in the support you can receive. It doesn't have to be an in-person get-together either, as Skype, FaceTime, or phone dates with your friends can often be enough. Book these in advance, so you will have things to look forward to in your busy schedule.

If you are able to share some of your struggles and vulnerabilities, you never know who might have an answer you didn't expect or a solution you didn't see; give them some credit, as hopefully you were friends with them for a reason.

Still, it must be said that sometimes it's hard to maintain friendships with friends who don't have kids. While it's important to maintain these connections, recognize, too, that you and your friends likely have different agendas, priorities, and timetables. To have deepening relationships with other families and couples, having shared experiences, especially with babies the same age as yours, is vital. Meeting up at the park, going to a kids' event, or even taking a walk together will help deepen bonds. We live in a transient world, however, and I can still remember the disappointment of finding out a family that we had connected with was moving hundreds of miles away, and thinking, "Hey, wait a minute! You can't do that—we were just starting to get along really well!" Still, it is always better to try to connect.

Online support groups can be a treasure trove of connection, inspiration, and useful advice, but social media can also be devastatingly judgmental and harsh. I have seen mothers crawl back into their caves of social isolation after being group-shamed on Facebook. Social media can be very unpredictable, so stay off sites where you know cruelty can be unleashed, and stick to groups where you truly get the support you need.

When You Feel That You Need Professional Help

If you get to the point where you're worried about your mental health, seeing a therapist or counselor can be tremendously helpful, especially if you're suffering from depression or anxiety. It can be a huge relief to get advice from a sympathetic, neutral ear who is there to discuss you and your needs and can offer suggestions and strategies that will help you feel better.

When You Are Depressed

Most of the mothers that I see with postnatal depletion will have depressive feelings, and a small number will have depression. While there is a significant overlap of symptoms of postnatal depletion and postnatal depression, there is a very small proportion of mothers I see with depression *without* postnatal depletion.

There are important differences between depressive feelings and clinical depression. Depressive feelings come and go and can be all consuming when you're engulfed in them, especially when you're tired and depleted. A mother with depressive feelings is often very aware of her thoughts and feelings. Depression, on the other hand, is a more constant state, and a depressed mother is often less aware of what's going on; it's more the people around her who really notice the changes in behavior, such as being withdrawn or anxious or lacking the usual spark.

A key governing point for a mother with depressive feelings is that she knows, essentially, that life is still good. A depressed mother has often lost connection with this. It is extremely important that a mother (and her partner) seek immediate help from a health-care practitioner experienced with postnatal mental health if there are concerns, talk, or thoughts of self-harm, or if there is an unrelenting pervasive feeling that life is not good and will never be what it was before the baby was born. Unfortunately, with clinical depression, you have much less insight into your feelings.

When You Have Anxiety

It is absolutely normal to be anxious about your brand-new baby. I think every mother I've ever spoken to has told me that they sometimes wake up in the middle of the night just to check that their baby is still breathing!

The words *anxiety* and *worry* are easily interchanged. Anxiety tends to be more an emotional experience that spills over into thoughts. Worry tends to be rooted in thoughts that spill over into our emotional world.

We can think of worry as the mental part of anxiety. Worry tends to be experienced in our heads; it is about specific realistic concerns or issues and their solutions, is more controllable and shorter lasting, and is accompanied by mild emotional distress. Anxiety tends to be experienced in "our bodies"; it is more diffuse, less realistic, and not solution oriented. It is harder to control and is longer lasting, and the emotional distress tends to be more severe.

Even though postnatal depression and postnatal anxiety are talked about synonymously in much of the medical research, I think it's important to separate them. Anxiety can occur with or without depression, but when it occurs with depression it is most commonly associated with minor or nonmelancholic depression. Postnatal anxiety disorders may be as common as depression and include generalized anxiety, phobias, obsessive-compulsive disorder, posttraumatic stress disorder, adjustment disorder, panic disorder, and agoraphobia.

I find there is a complex interplay among the various factors that lead to maternal anxiety. It can be particularly after the birth of a first child; the novelty, while special, is accompanied by feelings of uncertainty and the mother's growing awareness of the enormous learning curve that she's now on. Some women may harbor unrealistic expectations that everything will be perfect, and they can feel great disappointment and disempowerment when idealism and realism collide and events fall somewhat short of their hopes.

As I mentioned earlier, our firstborn, Felix, was quite an unsettled baby in the first year; he cried a lot and didn't sleep much. I remember the anxiety that Caroline and I experienced and how at 3:00 a.m. our anxieties could quickly spiral into a cascade. Even with all my medical knowledge and experience in a neonatal unit, as a father it was difficult not to worry. We can look back at this now with greater understanding, insight, perspective, and even gratitude that our own personal experience gives us empathy for what most, if not all, new mothers go through.

If, however, you find that everything triggers anxious thoughts and feelings and that anxiety is your default mode—especially if situations that you'd normally find relaxing or enjoyable, such as catching up with a friend for an afternoon coffee, are now causing you anxiety and worry—then you should seek help.

There are two conditions in which micronutrient deficiencies can lead to severe anxiety and an inability to manage stress, so it's worth knowing about them.

PYRROLE DISORDER

Pyrrole disorder is a "zinc-wasting" condition that affects about 10 percent of the population. Pyrroles are formed as part of a glitch that can occur when the body is breaking down and recycling hemoglobin, the protein that transports oxygen to your red blood cells. The body eliminates this partly metabolized dysfunctional hemoglobin unit, called a pyrrole, through the kidneys. The problem is that the pyrrole molecule latches on to zinc and vitamin B_6, and they are excreted together in the urine.

You already learned that zinc and vitamin B_6 are vitally important not only in regulating immune function and digestive health but also in maintaining healthy balances of brain neurotransmitters. Low levels will affect the brain chemical GABA (gama-aminobutyric acid), which is what helps slow down and soothe the brain, especially when it's getting overactive. (Valium and all the benzodiazepines treat anxiety by working on the GABA receptor in the brain.) More anxiety begets more pyrroles, which then exacerbates further anxiety through zinc and B_6 loss.

How to Test for Pyrrole Disorder

A simple urine test looking for normalized HPL (hydroxyhempyrolin) will show if you have pyrroles. A normal range is 0 to 10 mcg/dL; borderline is 10 to 15 mcg/dL; and anything over 15 mcg/dL is worth treating.

How to Treat Pyrrole Disorder

Large doses of zinc picolinate (40 to 75 mg) and vitamin B_6 (50 to 125 mg), as well as P5P (or pyridoxal-5-phosphate, which is activated vitamin B_6) (25 to 75 mg) and vitamin C (2 g) are the standard daily protocol. With more severe cases, if the HPL is around or above 50 mcg/dL, then biotin (500 mcg), vitamin E (400 IU), and gamma linoleic acid (1 to 2 g) in the form of evening primrose oil or borage oil are added to the daily routine. Most patients have a dramatic improvement after only one to two weeks, with full benefit usually taking place after one month.

I will typically do a course of treatment for three months with review. If you feel your stress/anxiety starting to snowball again, you can restart the zinc and vitamin B_6 protocol and you should feel better within a week or two. Some people need longer-term treatment, but this should only be done in conjunction with an experienced practitioner because there is some concern over the potential harms of long-term high-dose vitamin B_6 supplementation.

METHYLATION

Undermethylation

Methylation is the process of transferring a methyl group (a single carbon) from one molecule to another. This transfer takes place in every cell millions of times each *second*. Every enzyme and every metabolic process in your body require methylation. Postnatally, methylation is vitally important in the processing and elimination of a number of toxins, and it helps regulate the brain chemicals that balance your mood and concentration.

If your body is good at methylation, no worries. If, however, you tend to be an undermethylator, you will have a more exaggerated reaction, biochemically, to environmental stressors. You would know this if you have seasonal allergies, for example, or poor pain tolerance, which are exacerbated but not caused by undermethlyation. You might also have reduced amounts of serotonin (the "happy" brain chemical) and dopamine (the "pleasure" brain chemical). People with lower levels of serotonin tend to be overanalyzers; with lower levels of dopamine, it's harder to problem-solve or take pleasure in the good and positive things that are happening to you and your loved ones. This, of course, doesn't automatically lead to anxiety or depression, but it tends to lead you into a more pessimistic outlook in general. Being stuck in a world of dark and negative thoughts can then send you down that slippery slope where anxiety and depression become palpable. Those who have low serotonin and low dopamine due to undermethylation usually suffer from hypercritical thinking and anxiety.

Overmethylation

With overmethylation, you don't tend to fluctuate between highs and lows; everything is more even keeled—leaving some people feeling emotionally flat. Higher levels of serotonin keep in check tendencies to overanalyze and dwell on details. Higher levels of dopamine reduce motivation, and even though someone may not be feeling lazy or unmotivated or uncaring about things just being good enough, it can *seem* like this from an observer's viewpoint.

How to Test for Overmethylation and Undermethylation

A blood test should be done to check the whole blood histamine (WBH). If the WBH is higher than 0.6 umol/L (70 ng/ml), this is suggestive of undermethylation; a WBH of 0.35 umol/L (40 ng/ml) or lower indicates overmethylation. If you are having active allergies at the time of the blood test, it can make this test hard to interpret. A more accurate test is a methylation profile, which looks at four different metabolites—S-adenosyl-L-methionine (SAMe), S-adenosyl-L-homocysteine (SAH), tetrahydrofolate (THF), and L-methylfolate—and their ratios.

How to Treat Overmethylation and Undermethylation

For undermethylation, I prescribe a regimen of zinc, vitamin B_6, P5P, and SAMe (a synthetic version of a molecule that helps normalize the speed of methylation within your body). It's important to balance zinc and the other micronutrients before starting SAMe, and this usually takes four to six weeks. Avoid vitamin B_9 in the form of folate or folic acid—it can make your methylation worse.

For overmethylation, treatment typically is with vitamins B_9, B_3, C, and a special type of vitamin B_{12} called cyanocobalamin. There are other minerals and micronutrients that may or may not be added, depending on the test results. Be warned that, often, anxiety can get worse at around week 2 or 3, with a sharp improvement around weeks 4 to 8. Full effects take about three to four months. This is due to a rebalancing effect of brain neurotransmitters and usually isn't problematic as long as a mother is aware it is only short-lived.

Although these nutrient regimes aren't so much a fix, they can have a very positive effect on improving brain functioning and speeding up the path to recovery. Couple these regimens with counseling or therapy and you can gain true and long-lasting results for your anxiety.

I see so many mothers who feel validated and grateful for the acknowledgment that they are not suffering alone, that, in fact, what they're going through is something that is both understandable and sometimes even predictable. I especially hear this from mothers who have older kids and who, having been through this before, feel they should be beyond this stage of exhaustion and anxiety but are instead stuck in a rut. It's much easier to move forward with confidence knowing that this process, as described by one of my moms, is like fixing potholes in the road. You end up feeling less worried about hitting a pothole and more confident in your ability and energy to move ahead.

FINDING THE FLOW STATE THAT LEADS TO HAPPINESS

Everyone wants to be happy, right? When I discuss happiness with my patients, what I steer the conversation toward is understanding the difference between *being* happy and *doing* happy.

Being happy is being contented in the present moment. *Doing* happy is incessantly questing for those things that we think *should* make us happy—this is where we've come unstuck as a society. Because *doing* is an active process, there is an implication that if only you try harder you can have (or buy) more happiness. *Being* happy, on the other hand, is purely an experience in the now.

In the late 1960s and early 1970s, under the guidance of University of Chicago professor Mihaly Csikszentmihalyi, the largest global happiness study was undertaken. What this groundbreaking study showed was that many of the factors that people had been striving for in search of happiness were not particularly relevant, including money (beyond a certain degree of comfort). Quite a finding since our entire capitalistic worldview is based on the notion that money equals happiness! Instead, the study found that the happiest people were the ones who had the most "peak experiences."

A peak experience must have a degree of newness about it, include a sense of discovery, and contain an element of being outside your comfort zone. It does not need to be monumental, but it does, according to Dr. Csikszentmihalyi, require you to be in a "flow state." When you are so engaged in a task at hand that you lose track of the time, you are in a flow state. It could be when you're deep in a conversation with a dear friend or when you're in a yoga class and concentrating fully on your breath and movement. It could be when you're gardening and are mindfully pulling out each and every weed. Many of the activities of motherhood can, in fact, be direct triggers into a flow state—cooking, playing and doing crafts with the kids, or singing and making music. Being creative in any capacity—including reading a story aloud to your children—helps you get into a flow state... and being in a flow state in turn helps stimulate even more creativity.

Scientists who have taken brain scans of people in flow have found that during a flow state the prefrontal cortex part of the brain becomes less active. This is the area of the brain that controls your inner critic and monitors impulse control; it is involved in your sense of self and self-awareness. When the prefrontal cortex quiets down, your decision-making and pattern-recognition abilities improve.

Actually, we have two distinct systems of processing information in our amazing brains—sort of like the devil and the angel sitting on opposite shoulders, whispering into our ears when we're trying to make important decisions. The devil is the rule-based explicit system and controls conscious awareness in the prefrontal cortex. The angel, or implicit system, involves skill and experience and is not consciously accessible—this is often described as lateral thinking, which many of us have experienced as an inner voice or intuition. (Carl Jung defined this intuition as "perception by the unconscious.") When you're in a flow state, your angel tells your rule-based prefrontal cortex to calm down, allowing your intuition to be more in control.

This is important because your brain really does want to rely on your intuition when you've just had a baby—it accounts for your sixth sense of just knowing what your baby needs and even being able to anticipate it. If you're depleted, though, your intuition can be totally skewed. And if you're stressed about anything, even when your depletion is cured, flow can also be disrupted. As soon as the depletion is addressed, you'll find yourself automatically clicking into flow, and you'll feel so much happier.

Being a mother is hard work—there is no way around that—but the ability to weave flow into the fabric of your busy days and nights will transform you from an "Okay, I'm down with this, I guess" kind of mom to an awesome and blissfully fulfilled mom. But when you are deeply depleted, the flow state is utterly disrupted. This means that you'll be mentally jumping from one concern to another rather than being fully attuned to the task at hand.

If the stress is related to the flow activity—let's say you're in the kitchen making dinner and you drop a plate of food on the floor and have to deal with the mess—then after doing some slow breathing in and out (or sighing), what can actually help you get back into the work flow is doing something simple that requires all your immediate attention. For example, you might leave the mess on the floor and turn your attention to chopping up some vegetables. Once the heat of the situation has cooled off and the "How clumsy am I" thoughts have dissipated, *then* you will be in a better space to clean up the mess. Because chopping vegetables is the kind of task in which you need to concentrate on what you're doing, it brings you right back to the present moment (and the actual chopping is usually very satisfying)! Before you know it, you're back in your cooking-induced flow.

With all other factors being equal, the more we are in a flow state, the more happiness we'll experience. I live in a part of Australia where I'm surrounded by people pursuing dense flow states—from surfing and skateboarding and communing with nature to attending yoga classes or going to concerts. (And, no, perhaps surfing is not on the to-do list of most overburdened and depleted moms I've met!)

When you have lots of work and family-life disruptions, it's not always easy to find the time or place for flow. I have taken a deep look at my life and have been surprised to see how flow can come from some unexpected places. For me, if I'm presented with an active task that contains an element of repetitiveness and an element of challenge, then this is likely to trigger flow. If I take the dog for a walk, I am just as likely to daydream as I am to get into flow, but if I go barefoot and actively look for birds in the sky and feathers on the ground, and pay specific attention to what flowers are out, then a flow state comes more easily. Yoga, thanks to its breathing exercises, is also a fantastic way for me to get into a flow state. Ditto for playing soccer with my boys, especially when we pretend we are in the World Cup final—imagination-type games with my kids do the trick, too. I was a fairly serious child and did not play a lot in the world of imagination, so it doesn't come easily or naturally to me, but it provides the challenge element I need to experience flow. In my home, we have buckets full of disassembled LEGO pieces, and once, the kids and I decided to build a LEGO soccer stadium. We used all the figurines for our soccer teams and different sections of the stadium for *Star Wars* Storm Troopers and Middle Earth characters. It took us a few weeks and countless hours, but what I remember most was how time flew and how dense a flow state that was. And I was playing with the kids! It was fantastic for all of us.

Why is this important? Because to be an awesome mom, you need to be happy, and to be happy, you need to have flow coming in and out of your life all the time. This is incredibly easy and happens to you all the time without you realizing it—you just need to be *present*.

The best way to get back into regular flow states is to know what your triggers are. It could be playing a game of tennis, reading an absorbing book, listening to certain types of music, dancing, meditating, being with certain friends and loved ones, shopping for clothes in your favorite store, or playing catch with your toddler. Think about all the activities, people, and events that have triggered flow in the past. I like to use music as a trigger. It reminds me of my world outside this current moment in time. And it always makes me happy.

ANNA'S REGIMEN

Anna was thirty-two with a two-year-old girl. Her energy and libido were very low, she was having terrible problems with her guy, and she was experiencing huge levels of relationship stress. The year before, she had been diagnosed with depression. The antidepressants she'd been taking helped with her depression but not her libido, and she was still so anxious and agitated that her therapist took her off the meds completely. Her stress was ruling her life and making her miserable.

What the Testing Showed

As I suspected, Anna's adrenal hormones were very low and her pyrroles were very high. She had low blood protein and low levels of vitamin B_{12}. She also had yeast and a bacterial overgrowth in her gut.

Anna's Protocol

I devised a regimen around nutrition, digestive supplements, and herbs to correct her gut problems. I put her on a three-month plan with a compounded formula for her pyrroles, with zinc, trace elements, and specific B vitamins, including vitamin B_{12}. She also took adaptogenic herbs—ashwagandha, ginseng, shatavari, and schizandra.

Three months later, her "sensitive stomach" was much better, as were her anxiety and agitation. Because she was in a much calmer and clearer thinking space, she was better able to engage with her therapist and address her relationship issues. She found she wasn't getting so easily triggered when it came to emotionally charged topics and was able to maintain a central feeling of peace.

CHAPTER 12

Recovering Your Self-Love

PRACTICING SELF-LOVE

At its essence, the road to recovering and rebuilding your emotional well-being can be described in three words: *practice self-love.*

What does that mean exactly? Well, it's the act of nurturing yourself and putting yourself *first*—even if, at times, this will seem more a symbolic act than a practical and useful one. It's what you hear in the safety demonstration every time you get on an airplane. If the oxygen masks drop, put yours on before you put one on your children. If you are struggling with the word *self-love,* that's okay. Some of my moms like to swap it with *self-care* or *self-compassion* instead.

In our modern society, women have been socialized to put the needs of others before their own. They can even be harshly judged for identifying and revealing their own needs. The sacrifices of the perfect loving woman and mother should go without reward and acknowledgment, according to a centuries-old stereotype. And, in fact, when a mother is stressed-out, overwhelmed, and unsupported, she is often not seen by those around her. To be a mother, she is told, requires total dedication and to be in a place of service and surrender. It is actually much easier to succumb to these pressures and end up in a place of self-loathing than it is to feel entitled to self-compassion and self-love. It is easier to be an unsupported martyr than it is to be a self-caring mother.

The opposite of self-love is self-neglect, and this is what I see the minute a new patient in the full throes of postnatal depletion walks into my clinic. New moms are the champions of self-neglect. They have been told so many times that "a mother should give *of* herself." That drives me crazy, and I always hasten to tell these new patients that whoever said that to them needs to cut it out!

Self-love is not just something you deserve—it's what you *need*! Your body made a baby—and now you need to take the time to honor what you've been through and to appreciate what your body knew how to do without your actively governing it. You are devoting your time to taking care of a little creature who is demanding around-the-clock care—pat yourself on the back and take the time for a massage that will get the kinks out of your neck and shoulders. Your body was zapped of nutrients while you were pregnant—you *deserve* to eat the best food possible. You are now a mother—you *deserve* to be thrilled that you have created your family.

Our society tells us that newborns result in blissfully happy mommies, and this leaves mommies who are struggling out of the picture. Add a lack of support, understanding, or realistic checkpoints about how to measure your progress as a mother, and you have a recipe for worsening depletion.

The path of motherhood, while long and arduous, should at least be paved with constant support, education, and honoring your amazing achievement as you nurture another person through the world. If the path feels more like a rocky, rutted, unpaved country road, it's not fair for you to be blamed when your "feet"—your natural abilities to cope with life stresses—aren't yet tough enough for the journey!

When I see my patients struggling, I explain that the best place to start the practice of self-love is by attending to the Four Pillars of Health: sleep, purpose, activity, and nutrition (if you need a refresher, see page 52).

Self-Love and Sleep

One of the best and most nurturing forms of self-love is to prioritize your sleep, which you learned how to do in chapter 8. This isn't just about getting enough sleep—it's about making your sleep-time environment as lovely as possible. Even if the baby's bassinet or crib is in your bedroom, or if you are cosleeping with your older children, your bedroom should be the room in your home reserved only for sleeping and making love. It should be the nicest, most comfortable, and most welcoming room for *you* in your home. It has to feel good, be uncluttered, and be decorated in a way that makes you happy and helps you relax.

Self-Love and Activity

With activity, practicing self-love is about moving your body correctly and taking care of it. Remember, you are not a beast of burden whose sole job it is to lug around kids, groceries, toys, and heavy bags of diapers. Once your child feels too heavy to carry, then he or she *is* too heavy to carry!

It's very important for you to prioritize time to do the things that make your body feel good. This isn't just about keeping your body healthy—it's about all the wonderful ways you can relieve physical tensions and promote physical relaxation. Whether you decide to go for long walks, take a yoga class, get a massage, or soak in a warm, deliciously scented bath, this active kind of self-love is about moving your body in a way that it likes to be moved and supported. When you physically relax, you automatically reduce mental tension and promote mental relaxation. Just don't overdo it. You're getting over being depleted, so if any form of exercise or movement is making you feel tired, either during or after the activity, then stop. Go slow. Start with a few minutes and gradually increase the time.

Self-Love and Nutrition

If it weren't so important, the self-neglect that often occurs around food would almost be comical. My patients who have older children tell me all the time about the hours they spend food shopping and then cooking up nutritious meals for their kids, made with love, only to see the frowns and hear the groans from their kids before half of what was on their plate ends up on the floor. In my family, we are lucky to have

Lenny, our dog (aka "the Hoover"), who over the years has been the happy recipient of countless food "accidents." Some depleted moms try to satisfy their own nutritional requirements from mouthfuls of cold leftovers gulped down while they're busy finishing up either the kitchen chores or the "we have to get into the car right now because we are late" daily school or activity runs.

Not only do children need to see the importance that we place on food, but they also need to see *you* placing that importance on what *you* eat—and how and when. They need to see *you* enjoying food that you know is healthy and to be doing so in a sharing and caring manner. This is very much part of our evolutionary heritage. Sitting down together as a family to enjoy a meal shared by all is your goal, and if you establish regular eating times for family meals when your children are very young, it will be much easier to keep this schedule as they grow older.

Self-Love and Purpose

The idea of practicing self-love around purpose can be the most challenging. One of the reasons has to do with our personal value systems. What we *think* we value may not actually be what we *truly* value, and this dichotomy can become an enormous blind spot or stumbling block for you.

For example, you might be someone who values having a neat and presentable home and have always spent a lot of your time and energy cleaning and scrubbing. What you may not realize is that the more superficial goal of having a clean house is a smokescreen for your need for some kind of immediate result and gratification for the way you spend your time. Setting small goals such as doing the dusting and immediately seeing the tangible results might make you feel like you have served a purpose—but what you really want is acknowledgment of how important you are to your loved ones. There will always be dust and messes to clean up; much more difficult is to have recognition for *you*—not your cleaning skills!

Part of establishing a healthy, nurturing new life is resetting the vicious vs. virtuous cycle. Here's an example of a vicious cycle: In an effort to be Supermommy, you put on a brave face and a nice new lipstick to go to your mommy group, even though you are nearly dropping with exhaustion. Once you're there, the other mothers, who all seem to know one another well and who've also gone through their own supreme effort to look good, start to "talk good." This means they'll be talking good about all the things that they are doing or have read or that their huge support network did for them, and they go on and on about all the projects they're undertaking and the flexibility they have from their jobs (if they work). Of course you're happy for them that things are going well, but comparing their fantastic situations with yours makes you want to drag yourself home and start crying because your "I'm a terrible mom/wife/provider" button got pushed. You wonder why you aren't doing or feeling what the talk-good mommies are. You wonder if you've made a terrible mistake about your career or where you live because you don't have the support network that they seem to. Then you realize that not only are you upset, but you're also starving, so you reach for whatever food is closest and easiest, and it's definitely not a nutritious or healthy option. Once you've devoured it, the temporary relief is replaced with remorse and, if you ate a lot of sugar or carbs, is quickly followed by plummeting blood sugar levels that leave you even more exhausted. But you're determined to push past all this, so you go on with your day even as the tears are lurking. You're operating so close to the edge that you yell at your baby for waking up too soon from a nap or for peeing all over the changing table, and you can't sleep because you feel so bad about everything that happened. The next day you wake up already exhausted, and that leaves the "I'm a terrible mom/wife/provider" button even more exposed than it was the day before. The vicious cycle starts again.

The reverse cycle here is called the virtuous cycle. This doesn't mean that you will never cry (it's okay when you do) or that you'll never question yourself (there's a lot to figure out!) or that you'll never wish that you had something that others do (it's impossible to know what your needs as a parent will be until you're doing it). But when you can set your cycle from vicious to virtuous, you are able to see those button-pushing moments and know that they are natural and do not mean that there is something wrong with the way that you are parenting. It means that you might go to a mommy meeting, hear all the other moms bragging, and remind yourself they're actually putting on a brave front, too, because of course their babies are just as time-consuming and exhausting to take care of as yours is. It means that you might see another family's impeccably kept home but be able to enjoy the fun that you had in your own home that led to it being a little messier. It means that when it seems like all the other moms are hanging out without you, you reach out, either to them or to someone already in your own life, and give yourself a taste of real connection rather than getting lost in the feeling of being alone. Your self-love has you surround yourself as best as you can with things, people, and activities that make you feel better (*not* worse) about yourself.

You don't want to find yourself falling into martyrdom, where you feel that you must sacrifice yourself and your needs in order to take care of your baby. This is easy enough to say but of course not necessarily easy to do. Women biologically are more driven toward a sense of order and can be seen as being more perfectionist than men. It can also follow that women are less likely to have an internal measuring stick to comfortably say "That's good enough" or "I can stop thinking about this now."

I see this phenomenon so often that I named it the Mother vs. Martyr Challenge. There is a big difference between a mother who when facing difficulties will try better and smarter and a mother who will only try harder. Trying harder to do the same thing without being happy with the results makes this mom a martyr. I very seldom see a mother who has not been trying hard enough—it's usually a mother trying *too* hard that's the problem. A mother who's trying too hard will spend all her time and energy doing tasks and jobs that leave her in a state of overload. If she remains in this state, she will totally wear herself out. What she's not doing, and should be doing, is spending some of her time simply in a state of just being, unpressured and calm.

Every decision in life has consequences—much like a sequence of falling dominoes—but it's possible to step in and break the chain if you don't like where things are going. Ultimately it is *you* who decides when to push that first domino.

It is worth really thinking about how you spend your time and seeing where the joy comes from. Is there any priority around those things that enrich your life? Does your need to have a spotless home come from the sense of calm that control and order can bring? Or is it purely out of a sense of obligation? Are there things that take up your time now that you don't get rewarded by? If yes, do you *have* to do them? Is there a way to share or delegate the responsibilities that are sucking out your energy without paying anything back?

It is important to reassess not only your priorities but also your goals, what you truly value, and what you feel your purpose is—because these are the things you want to model for and impart to your children as they grow older. One commonly suppressed value my patients often discuss with me is creativity. Due to time and energy constraints, these moms are too busy to connect with their creative selves, and they push down their own goals and purpose (such as writing, music, and art), which is a shame because it would make them (and, ultimately, their children) feel a lot better to have the much-needed outlet.

Everyone needs to feel that they're good at something—because everyone *is* really good at something. This could be writing an award-winning screenplay, being a beloved teacher, nurturing a lovely garden, or figuring out a recipe for the tuna casserole your kids adore. Purpose doesn't mean material success—it means personal satisfaction, being a good and loving person, and sharing your love and goodness with the important people in your life. Always remember that you are unique and wonderful and the best mom for *your* child. That's what's really important in life.

CHAPTER 13

Recovering Your Relationship with Your Partner and with Your Libido

When Chief Red Cloud, leader of the Oglala Lakota tribe, became a father, he went outside, threw his hands skyward, and said, "Now I can become a full man."

If a father is involved early on, during the birth and those early weeks following birth, studies show that he can become much more hormonally linked to his child: his testosterone can actually decrease by as much as one-third after the birth. Prolactin, a hormone that we almost exclusively associate with breastfeeding, can increase in these same fathers, and this seems to translate to a greater responsiveness to their babies' crying.

Becoming a parent is an incredible experience for dads as well as for moms—challenging them to grow and to explore their long-held ideas about masculinity and manhood. Both parents need to acknowledge that having a baby is a major life event that can place an astronomical amount of strain on a relationship. Men not fully understanding their role as fathers and not often having grown up with a learned vocabulary and understanding of a woman's, mother's, and partner's needs can find themselves feeling very isolated. As the fallback position is to be provider and protector for the family, many men spend more time at work and as a result become more disconnected and distant from their partners.

After recovering from your postnatal depletion and feeling like yourself again, these issues around the health of your relationship invariably come up. If there were fractures present in the relationship before the birth, they can open up into seismic chasms after the baby's arrival.

One important issue I see constantly has to do with relationship stress and conflict. Many recovering mothers hit a road block in terms of the "relationship satisfaction" they are experiencing with their partners.

Even with the healthiest couples, their relationship satisfaction is at its lowest eighteen months after the birth of a child. Studies I have read over the years have claimed that 13 percent of couples call it quits at this stage or earlier, by either divorce or separation. (In Australia, the median age at divorce is 44.8 years for men and 42.2 years for women, with 47 percent of divorces involving children under eighteen.) Of those who stay together, 25 percent describe their relationship as being "in distress." Furthermore, 92 percent of couples describe a gradual increase in conflict after having a baby.

What's key here is that, if not addressed and supported, these pressures and problems can cause satisfaction with your partner to erode over time. Some relationships can't last due solely to incompatibility issues, but I believe they are in the minority. Often, relationships break up due to lack of support, lack of resources or tools to deal with the issues, and financial stressors.

But it's never too late to start improving your relationship. Just as relationships can slowly worsen over time, they can also slowly improve. Small changes can make big differences. What's most important is how you and your partner manage your decision-making process and how well you can communicate about it. You can't and shouldn't try to avoid problems—they're a part of being a parent, of being in a relationship, and of life in general!

THE RELATIONSHIP DYNAMICS THAT CONTRIBUTE TO DISSATISFACTION

When you look at modern relationships, there have never been so many demands and expectations put on couples as there are today. We expect ourselves and our partners to be providers, coparents, best trusted friends, passionate lovers, successes in their own fields, healthy and good-looking individuals, and unconditional sources of love and support. If your expectations aren't met, there's a tendency to jump to negative conclusions about the state of the relationship, your partner's state of mind, and his or her motives.

The honeymoon, or passionately-in-love, phase of a relationship typically lasts about two years. As we move from this romantic love to a more mature love, we have to start learning to share our vulnerabilities. To do this, we need to learn how to embrace the notion of mature love over romantic love and find a balance between security and passion.

It may be tempting to fixate on your partner's habits because that takes the focus away from having to confront your own fears, which a shift in your relationship can bring up. Which habit drives you the craziest? Does he always squeeze the toothpaste tube from the middle? Does he hum when he's driving? Does he slurp his soup? Does he forget to call when he says he will?

These little habits that are annoying yet trivial in the larger scope of your life can suddenly become big problems when you are exhausted and depleted—they grow to symbolize that you feel you're not being listened to. It's often very hard to communicate how you feel about these things, yet we expect others to know just how vital they are. No one can read your mind. Expecting your partner to know what you need without *your* having to figure it out yourself falls into the realm of magical thinking!

In the midst of a tough parenting moment, whether it's a long train of sleepless nights, a difficult behavioral period, or an acute crisis of some kind, it's common to feel isolated from your partner. This can be especially hard to cope with because it feels like you two are supposed to be in it together, and yet you may react very differently to the same situation. If so, you may find thoughts like "If you truly loved me..." or "No one understands..." or "You are holding me back..." come flooding into your head. It can be very tricky to manage this when you are already in such a vulnerable state without outside help.

IMPROVING YOUR COMMUNICATION SKILLS

What distinguishes happy from unhappy marriages is not what kind of positive experiences you have together but how you *interpret* them. The best way to improve your relationship is not to have more positive experiences but to decrease the negative ones. Key to this is learning how to communicate productively about everything in between. That starts with getting better at stating your needs and expectations.

Good communication is at the heart of all thriving relationships, and it involves the capacity to give another person an accurate picture of how you feel. When we don't communicate, we act out in toxic ways—through avoidance, excuse making, withdrawal, depression, and/or anger.

A common scenario with couples who aren't communicating well centers, not surprisingly, on the frequency of having sex; often he wants more and she wants hardly any. He feels rejected; she feels guilty. He feels like a failure, undesired and helpless. It is common for the father to having feelings of jealousy when he sees the amount of loving attention the baby receives. It can be challenging for him to even identify this jealousy, much less figure out how to handle it, and this can leave the mother feeling alone, unsupported, and objectified. He feels he is never good enough and that nothing he does is right; she feels stressed, like she is doing everything alone, and is frustrated by his needs. He feels his need for love and connection is interpreted by her as being wrong, demanding, primitive, selfish, childish. She feels she can't relax, can't let go, and can't get the intimacy and touch she truly desires. Both feel very alone and frustrated, and resentment starts to build, eventually leading to either passive-aggressive behavior or an explosive, angry conflict.

But these issues can be avoided if you set aside a time to talk openly and honestly about your feelings, fears, and doubts. While I am no expert in relationships, I have worked with numerous relationship therapists and done extensive research on this topic because it's so important for my patients—I've seen firsthand how the cold war between couples via misunderstanding and miscommunication further stresses already depleted mothers. Every couple deserves and needs a relationship based on honesty and empathy in which each is fully able to enrich the life of the other through love and attentiveness to each other's needs.

Without wanting to overgeneralize, I have noticed that men tend to have much more single focus with attention and efforts, whereas women tend to have much more diffuse awareness. The male brain is more wired to task-oriented work and mathematical logic than to the world of emotions and openness. Men often do not have as much experience as women do with expressing their thoughts, fears, and feelings—or listening well without wanting to jump in and instantly decide they are the only ones with solutions—so they have to learn on the job, often in the heat of the moment, about communication issues that don't necessarily come naturally. If what you need from your partner is an open space to talk without feedback, try starting the conversation by explicitly asking for that.

Moreover, men tend to be more internally motivated when it comes to tasks and tend to judge themselves more from internal standards, whereas women tend to be more perfection motivated and judge themselves more from external standards, such as what their friends might think. This is a source of misunderstanding, as assumptions are made around these "standards."

Without proper resolution, conflicts can linger and grow from small annoyance to intense anger. This isn't always a bad thing, *if* your anger is used to give you the energy and motivation to create change. But anger and frustration must be tempered by compassion—which will be lacking if there is unkind judgment, comparisons with others, and denial of responsibility.

Resolving conflicts must start with reconnection, whether from a place of intimacy or from sharing something you love to do together, such as watching a movie. It is like hitting the reset button. From that place of reconnection, you can start a new cycle of talking openly without fear of censure and truly listening to each other. Expressing your vulnerability and fears is a great way to start—all new parents have these feelings, and being able to admit it helps mitigate them in a loving way.

When a couple is in a state in which they are more connected than in conflict, they can then start the challenging but amazingly liberating work of exploring their deepest needs. Don't start up a "needs conversation" when your partner is focused on something else. Schedule a quiet time to have it—this really works!

How Men Should Frame the Questions

What you want to strive for is talking less and communicating more. Don't take criticism personally. Listen without interruption and refrain from being wholly solutions oriented. (This can be very hard for men to do.) This kind of gentle empathy will help your partner open up. Try these helpful comments:

- Tell me more…
- Help me understand that better…
- What else would you like me to do?

Validate your partner's feelings, even if you don't totally agree with them. Don't say things like "How can you feel that way? It's ridiculous." It might be ridiculous to you, but not to your partner! Expressing gratitude even for the smallest things can go a long way toward making your partner feel loved and needed. End your conversation by reaffirming how much you love and care for each other.

How to Tell a Man What You Need

Women often don't realize (or they forget) that most men really do want to contribute and play an active role in raising the baby, but they are better able to help when they feel they have specific tasks or duties that belong to them. You want to make him feel not only that you are honoring his contribution but that this will in turn satisfy your needs as a mother and partner. Essentially, men do really well with specific suggestions around how to give you the support you need—they want to provide solutions!

Remember that a man will easily misinterpret suggestions, corrections, ideas for improvement, and constructive criticism as "complaints," and once a man hears a complaint, he will get defensive and start to detach. Do your utmost to listen to him without interruption so you can keep the conversation flowing. Here are some conversational guidelines:

- Be very specific about your needs, using language he will understand. Let him know how it makes you feel and why it is important. For example, say, "I need you to be home by 5 p.m. twice a week so you can pick up groceries, prepare dinner, and clean up and bathe the baby. Your doing this will give me two hours of calm where I won't feel overwhelmed and stressed. I would feel more supported when you do this." This is not a demand but a request—very different from you angrily saying, "You need to be home more and do more. I've had enough and I need a night off!"
- Avoid demands whenever possible. The only two responses someone has to a demand are to grudgingly submit or rebel, which leads to criticism and judgment. Saying "You have to" is less likely to work than saying "If you chose to..."
- Asking a man to *provide* is more inspiring for him than asking him to *do*. Try asking open-ended questions, such as "What would you need so you can provide this for me?" Or "Is there a particular way I can show my appreciation for you giving me this?" Wait for his answer—you may be surprised at what he says!
- No interruptions! Let him speak.
- Think before you blurt out any judgments or overanalysis. You may change your mind about the topic later but can't unsay what was said.
- Even your partner, who knows you well and loves you, is not a mind reader. No one can tell what you are feeling and thinking unless you express your needs and thoughts in precise language. If you feel anxious or depressed, you need to say so. If this is difficult for you, professional counseling might be a valuable addition to your postdepletion arsenal, because a neutral party can make it easier for you to talk openly.

Becoming a parent is a life transformation, and you are not the same person as before. Wanting life to return to the way it was won't work; it will never happen. You and your partner need to be aware of this transformation and be ready to adjust to the new. Moms also need to trust their partners. You have to learn to let go of your need to control and embrace the fact that your partner will feed and change and cuddle the baby differently from you, and that's okay. Letting go of control can make a mother feel more vulnerable initially, but there is usually such a sense of relief once the apprehension is worked through, and this often leads to her partner becoming much more involved in baby care.

DAD TALK IS IMPORTANT, TOO

For men, becoming a father is a peak emotional experience with no equal. Because it is such a powerful event, it will bring up all kinds of feelings, many of which may be new or previously not felt in such depth. And, of course, it will also bring up many questions and doubts.

I wish we lived in a society in which our elders could sit us down and tell us what to expect from fatherhood, delineating our role so we could reap the rewards of this guidance. But there is not a lot of information, dialogue, or support for fathers-to-be. We essentially learn on the job, with all the joy and the pitfalls that this brings.

Since many men over-rely on their partners for emotional support and are not used to or skilled in confiding in or getting support from others, the challenge (and the solution) for them lies in making changes in their emotional routine. These men often unwittingly rate the closeness of their relationship by how much intimacy is occurring. When we have a partner who is struggling or exhausted, we can feel our connection weaken, especially as our vulnerabilities come easily to the surface, leaving us feeling threatened. It's not easy to process all this, but now more than ever is the time when men must be solid in their vulnerabilities and put aside many of their needs, even while asking themselves, "Where do I go for support?" "Where do I go for information?" "Who will help me if I am confused or overwhelmed?"

Sometimes becoming a mother can make you realize the work you were doing before no longer has the same meaning for you, or it can make you love your work even more and feel more passionate about it. Being a mother can make you more creative and yearn for time for more self-expression. Be ready for these thoughts and feelings. Look at them as an invitation to go beyond, and use them to figure out what you truly want to do. Do *not*, however, let this shift in your thinking create a rift between you and your partner. If you're having trouble communicating how your thinking has shifted—and this is understandable because this crossroad is confusing for all involved and needs considerable care and

Without guidance, many men can respond to these changes either by needing more from their partner (which is very difficult if their partner is struggling with depletion) or by distancing themselves with work or hobbies. As mentioned previously, studies show that the rates of postnatal depression are at the 10 percent mark among fathers, which is close to the 13 to 16 percent rates that occur in mothers.

Postnatal depression among fathers is unique in the world of depressions; it doesn't have the typical risk factors, such as a previous history of depression, that you would see with other types of depression. Not surprisingly, the main risk factor for a father getting depression is whether or not the mother has depression. This telling fact shows that if mothers aren't coping, then fathers will have a hard time coping as well.

I blame no man when a family is struggling, and I understand how difficult it is to get understanding or support when a new baby upends the harmony of the household. Even when things are going well, being parents in today's society is loaded with minefields (and mind fields!). Fatherhood requires a different thinking and a different type of logic and agenda. No longer does the question "What would I like to do right now?" have much relevance. Instead, it needs to shift to "What do I need to do for my family right now?"

sensitivity to be properly dealt with—you might find that professional guidance and expertise will enable you to better express your feelings.

RECOVERING YOUR LIBIDO

A healthy, thriving libido is not so much a *goal* as it is the end result of a body and life fully in harmony. The transition from romantic love to mature love—the kind of love that allows for a successful transition from a purely romantic relationship with your partner to a family-based relationship—is not something that necessarily comes naturally. Before your first baby is born, it's easy to think that you can handle any shifts in your relationship. But things change a lot once children have actually arrived, and all bets are off if you're depleted! It's really hard to get in the mood for sex when your previously candlelit boudoir has become Baby Central, crammed with a bassinet and crib and all the baby paraphernalia that seem to multiply overnight.

Let's Talk about Sex

Sex is a huge part of the complicated dynamic between a couple after the baby comes along. Your role has shifted from lover to mother, and these are two archetypes that clash—or at least find it difficult to coexist. This, obviously, is confusing not only for a partner, but also for a woman who's in overwhelm as she travels over new terrain without a compass to help her navigate the way forward.

It can be very difficult for your partner to accept a new role, not just with the baby but also in how you see each other. Your love is going to shift, whether you think it will or not. Many new moms have conflicting feelings of guilt for not tending to their partner's needs because the baby's needs are so demanding. If that's you, you might feel completely irritated by your partner's needs, which strike you as supremely selfish at this time, especially if he's jealous of your breasts now that your baby has the monopoly on them. And if you've lost your libido, then sex may seem like something to schedule in solely for your partner's sake—not for your pleasure as well. To make the transition from partners to parents, both of you need to be able to communicate openly and offer each other support and patience as you sort through your needs and desires.

When your sexual needs aren't addressed, I often see a kind of numbness that sets in, with both partners giving up. This usually occurs after a downward spiral within a year or two after the birth of your baby—especially if this is a second child, which places an extra burden on an already burdened relationship. This is one reason so many couples break up during this time frame, with mothers initiating the breakup 75 percent of the time.

Libido isn't just about sex. It's about maintaining that delicate balance between biochemical/hormonal drives and social/emotional feelings. It can be mysterious and magical or painful and relationship breaking.

I think that's because libido is one of the hardest topics for my patients to discuss. Sexual activity and sexual interest (or lack of) is often a huge issue for depleted moms. I know how hard this is because talking about such an intimate topic of sex and sexual urges can be deeply uncomfortable at the best of times. Factor in an exhausted, sleep-deprived mom and this conversation can be even more difficult.

I see so much guilt written on my patients' faces that it's often heartbreaking. They truly love their partners. They had a thriving, mutually satisfying physical relationship before the baby came along. They don't want their partner to feel left out or neglected even if they are living with the same sense of separation and alienation that the new father might be experiencing. But they can only handle so much, and when postnatal depletion is in charge, their libido and ability to manage their part in a relationship that was once seemingly so easy are often the first things to be shoved to the back of the emotional closet to be dealt with later. This can be compounded for new mothers who are coming to grips with the physical changes to their bodies that were brought on by pregnancy and delivery. These moms often feel, especially if it takes a while for them to shed weight and restore their old energy, that their own bodies have failed them. This is not exactly a recipe for romance!

For most new moms, sexual desire typically returns around six to seven weeks after giving birth. How strong a woman's libido is—and how on par it is with what it was before pregnancy—is influenced by the difficulty level of the birth and recuperation as well as how much support and understanding her partner is providing as a new father. What I have found is that many fathers who are in the delivery room for the birth of their babies tend to report higher levels of sex drive and feelings of closeness with their partners in the months after the birth. It's not a turnoff to them at all. The real top sex-drive killers are fatigue, the baby's sleep habits, and lack of time. No surprises there!

But take heart: though your libido may have plummeted thanks to hormonal and other physiological changes, this can quickly be remedied. And once you are aware of how your relationship with your partner has shifted, you can both address your fears and figure out how to manage them together.

The Physiological Reasons Why Having a Baby Wreaks Havoc on Your Libido

In scientific literature, libido is often defined as a fluctuating state of sexual motivation comprising four main components: arousal, desire, award, and inhibition. Arousal and desire have to do with how our body communicates to our brain via an interacting network of biochemistry, hormones, and our nervous system. Reward and inhibition occur purely in the brain and have to do with past experiences, emotional expectations, stress levels, and fear. All these components are responsible for changing your libido level.

Physical Recuperation after the Birth

If you gave birth vaginally, there will be bruising, soreness, and numerous microabrasions (tiny tears). There are often large tears, too, either from an episiotomy or from the birth itself. Whether you have stitches or not, a lot of healing needs to happen. The cervix has to close and the uterus has to return to its normal state; as it does, there will be a vaginal discharge called lochia, which slowly lessens over a six-week period.

The pelvic floor after the battlefield of pregnancy and birth will often not return to its original state for up to three months—something new mothers certainly know. If you gave birth via C-section, it can take up to six weeks to recover, and sex should be avoided for at least four weeks or until your doctor gives you the go-ahead.

Most of my new moms report that they resume having sex after about six to eight weeks. In 2013, a study published in the *British Journal of Obstetrics & Gynaecology* stated that 41 percent of first-time mothers had had full vaginal sex by the time the baby was six weeks old. But every new mom is different, of course. If you are feeling sensitive in the vaginal area, lubrication can be very helpful, especially as vaginal dryness is very common in the first two to three months following delivery. If you find that sex is painful, you should see your doctor right away to figure out if there is an infection or if the healing of vaginal tears hasn't occurred correctly, causing areas of constriction and tightness.

Being sexual and sensuous doesn't mean full-penetration intercourse has to happen. I think it's important for mothers to venture slowly back into sexual life without a goal-oriented agenda. Again, open communication with your partner is essential.

Altered Hormone Levels

Another simple cause for a diminished libido is hormonal. When you're pregnant, your female hormones greatly increase. Many women enjoy lovemaking up until their ninth month, and some find it easier to orgasm. Others are physically uncomfortable due to the extra weight/position of the baby and prefer to postpone sexual activity until after the birth.

After the baby is born, as you learned in chapter 6, your hormones (estrogen, progesterone, and cortisol) plummet. Until they return to normal levels, you may find it difficult to even consider sex because your body is being told that it needs to recuperate and restore—and sex isn't part of this recovery! With low levels of progesterone and cortisol, a mother is going to feel tired, possibly vulnerable, and not necessarily in a state of feeling great about herself. Combined with increased levels of oxytocin and dopamine from breastfeeding and being with the baby, she will likely experience a lower-than-usual sex drive and less need for connection with her partner and the outside world.

How to Test for Hormonal Causes of Low Libido

Your doctor, naturopath, or health-care provider can test your saliva to determine high or low cortisol, low DHEAs, and low testosterone. Any or all of these hormonal levels can cause and/or contribute to low libido.

How to Treat Low Libido Due to Hormones

See chapter 6 for information on how to treat low hormone levels.

The Libido Mismatch

In addition to your hormones needing time to adjust, you also have to contend with a basic difference between men's and women's sex drives. Nature is pretty smart. Its goal is perpetuation of the species. So Nature has worked out ideal levels of sexual behavior that will ensure enough reproduction so our species lives on.

What does this mean for you? Well, it means that part of Nature's design is that men, thanks to their generous levels of testosterone, have a constant interest in sexual activity. Women, on the other hand, tend to get more interested in sex around the time of month when they're ovulating and their estrogen and progesterone levels are higher. This biological difference in the libido levels of men and women is called the libido mismatch.

Interestingly, men's libido may go *up* during stressful times—this is Nature's innate mechanism for encouraging a man to pass on his genes before he gets "taken out" by whatever is causing the stress. For women, the opposite is usually true. Back in our ancestors' time, pregnancy and childbirth put a woman at huge risk, so getting pregnant made a woman more vulnerable to getting "taken out." If danger is lurking, the last thing you're going to think about is sex—blame your hormones for that one!

If you couldn't discuss the libido mismatch and your partner's wanting sex a lot more than you do *before* the baby was born, it's going to feel impossible to have this conversation when you're depleted. It can cause tremendous confusion for you both.

You need to find a way to discuss your new roles and the fact that spontaneous romantic love is not likely to happen during the recovery stage and even during the first few years with the baby. Your intimacy needs to be planned and scheduled now, and the definition of intimacy needs to change to include not merely sexual penetration but other forms of sex and sensual intimacy. If you can incorporate a sense of play, too, then sex is more likely to become a deeply satisfying place you go, not just an act you do.

Breastfeeding

One libido-killer that is rarely discussed or understood is breastfeeding. Breastfeeding increases the release of prolactin and decreases the release of estrogen and other sex hormones, including testosterone. The more you are breastfeeding, the less fertile you will be and the lower your sexual desire. This makes evolutionary sense. Once your baby is six months of age and able to eat solid food, you won't need to breastfeed as much, so fertility levels will go back up and your libido will also return—if you're not depleted. Deciding when to stop breastfeeding is an individual decision that results from the weighing of pros and cons, and I don't think that your libido level should be one of the factors considered.

Another libido reducer thrown into the mix is oxytocin. Breastfeeding and skin-to-skin contact with the baby saturate the oxytocin part of the brain, so the mother does not have the drive to get more oxytocin from her partner. She may still crave it but more in an emotional, nonphysical sense. Oxytocin is also what's triggered and released when you fall in love. So, to simplify a lot of complicated biochemistry, if your body has to choose between the needs of a breastfeeding baby and those of an eager-beaver partner, whom do you think is going to get chosen? Your baby, of course!

For a woman to be receptive to sex, all four aspects of libido—desire, reward, arousal, and inhibition—have to be in balance. Thanks to oxytocin, breastfeeding moms have a unique intimacy with their little one—not a sexual intimacy, of course, but rather a special bond that satisfies both desire and reward from a wholly new place. That is the biological imperative of survival of the species in action. This can mean that the intimacy—and the kind of intimacy—that a breastfeeding mother craves is not the sexual intimacy that she and her partner typically enjoy.

It's also not unreasonable, due to frequent breastfeeding, and possibly lots of cuddles with their children, for mothers to feel "all touched out." This means their need for touch and intimacy has been met and surpassed by children in a nonsexual way, and there's just nothing left over for a loving partner who wants some of that intimacy, too. With so much oxytocin already expressed, some mothers can even feel somewhat invaded and just need physical space. This can be confusing and alienating for a partner who quite understandably feels hurt and rejected as a result of something that doesn't make a lot of sense to him.

Sexual Inhibition

Yet another player in loss of libido is sexual inhibition. There are usually two reasons for this. Obviously, libido drops for both partners immediately after having satisfying sex. But it can also plummet because of a stressful life event (such as childbirth and taking care of a newborn while being depleted). It's not uncommon for a new mom to be dismayed by her postbirth figure, with a belly area still stretched out from the baby as well as a vagina that feels forever changed—and she's likely fretting about when and how she's going to return to her less saggy and more toned self. Simply not feeling sexy can increase inhibition.

Sexual inhibition occurs when the thinking part of your brain overrides the desire-seeking part. When out in public and surrounded by others, most people, for example, will inhibit feelings of arousal and refuse to entertain any acts coming out of that arousal. Overcoming sexual inhibition requires a combination of being in a relaxed state and being open to starting a new chapter with your partner. This is called reframing, but I much prefer the idea of starting a new chapter because it gives you a sense of moving forward to something new and yet to be explored.

A New Kind of Sex

What is clear from the research is that women want sex as much as men, but it is not the same kind of sex. Part of the evolution of mature love is also a maturing of the vocabulary of what sex means. Sex no longer becomes something that couples do but rather a place they go together. It becomes a container of both time and space, which a couple can enter together to explore and play. Imagine this place as your own personal Garden of Eden, where you can unite in bliss without all the hang-ups of the world pressing on your shoulders!

The lust-driven, spontaneous sex that childless couples thrive on will likely not happen nearly as frequently. With children in the house, sex may need to become planned. Each partner can now learn more about the intimate space with each other. Often the mother may not know herself fully in this space given everything that has changed, so it becomes an opportunity for joint exploration, support, and growth.

In other words, instead of fighting these changes, try being open to them. You may be surprised to find your relationship in a much richer place when exploring the new dynamic becomes the focus. This can only happen when there is a willingness from both parties to look for mutually pleasing solutions. If sexual needs aren't addressed or are left to simmer, then the relationship stays in the haphazard dance of blame and shame that many couples know only too well. A father needs to grow into his new role knowingly, kindly, and selflessly, but he should also feel that he can express any frustrations or hurt candidly and without fear of censure from his partner. See what compromises can be worked out. As you learned already, these are conversations that must be had, preferably when you're not keeling over in exhaustion!

Most of all, you need to stress over and over again that the presence or absence of sex does not indicate anything about a man's desirability or lovability. Hopefully, you will both soon get back into sexual sync, and all will be well—in and outside of the bedroom.

My suggestion is to create a time and a place where you and your partner can meet intimately as two adults. Schedule this just as you'd schedule a doctor's appointment. This is your very necessary playtime, and just like playtime for kids, it's not meant to be goal oriented. It's not about needing to have a mind-blowing orgasm—it's more about regularly meeting for intimate play that makes you both happy.

Conclusion

Through my journey as a doctor and as a father, through my exposure to so many experiences and people in my life, and through my research on postnatal depletion, I feel I have in some way been given a "download" to share. The result has been this book—an amalgamation of my life's work with many of the insights about postnatal depletion that came to me in the wee hours when I was doing much of my research for this book. I feel blessed and grateful to now have a healthy family, and through our struggles, I feel that my purpose in life is to be a leading voice in the revival of motherhood as an honored and respected path—a genuine heroine's journey.

My deepest motivation for writing this book has been to help mothers understand why they are depleted and also to help them understand how our modern society has allowed this to happen. I am honored to be a guide and education source for mothers on the road from depletion to repletion, then to recovery. Lucky me to have collaborated with many amazing thinkers and wellness-centric health practitioners to make this book as comprehensive as possible.

Through a medical starting point with testing, supplementation, and the support of health-care professionals, I am seeing mothers recover from the upheaval of postnatal depletion and become transformed every single day. Their energy returns, they can sleep well again, their hormones and emotions are back in check, and their brains are working better than ever. This allows them to find their voice and be the people they want to be—not just mothers to their babies but contributing members to their communities and the future. What I call *Mothermorphosis*!

When you realize that you no longer have to accept your depleted state as inevitable and unyielding, you will, I have no doubts, regain your strength. I am passionate about empowering mothers around the world to be both connected and educated so that they can make the best possible decisions for themselves and their families. This is a new way of motherhood in which the wisdom of the ancients becomes the medicine of the future.

When the Dalai Lama famously said at the 2012 Vancouver Peace Summit that "the world will be saved by the western woman," he was nearly right! The world will, in fact, be saved by the Western *mother.* By mothering the mother, and as mothers unite, the sisterhood of support and knowledge can be reestablished, and mothers can again find the mentorship that was present in our communities (as you read in chapter 1!) for thousands of years. As a society, we can then truly heal from the ground up. And there is much healing that needs to happen. By understanding and treating postnatal depletion, we can push back against the misinformation and the lack of support from previous generations, if only to make things easier and better for our children, as they will for theirs.

This is not a call to arms—but more a call to *be in* arms!

As a man, it's clear to me the world can heal only if women are united, as men do not inherently have the ability to form and unite communities. In the celebration of the differences between men and women lies the solution to much of the social disharmony of our society. Women, after all, are the ones who give birth—yet our society and especially our medical system treats expectant mothers like men and expects them to deny their depletion and just get on with it. Time for that to change.

I feel incredibly optimistic about the future. I've seen the astonishing ability of our bodies to heal and our souls to forgive. As we become more conscious as parents, we can be more honest about the world that we live in, and by reducing the overwhelming maze of daily choices and reducing the background noise of societal expectations, we can be much clearer in our intentions, too. What is most valuable is right in front of us, and through our children we can truly experience contentment.

I look forward to supporting you back to wellness.

APPENDIX A

Jump-Start Your Recovery

This overview will help you jump-start your recovery from postnatal depletion.

THE SIX-WEEK ACCELERATOR PLAN

Follow these guidelines for six weeks.

1. *Get Good Sleep*

- Go to bed as early as you can. This is number one on this list for a reason and is not negotiable! For all the tips you need, go back to chapter 8.
- Nap when you can.

2. *Take Good Supplements*

Basic Supplements to Take Every Day	
DHA	2 g
Zinc	25 mg
Iron	30 mg
Multimineral with calcium	
Choline	100 to 200 mg
Multiactivated B groups	
Ashwagandha (I prefer the Organic India brand)	two 500 mg capsules twice a day

3. *Have a Restorative Therapy Session Every Week*

- Go to a gentle or restorative yoga class, or make an appointment with an acupuncturist. Ask someone to take care of the baby for a couple of hours. You really need these sessions to help you relax and to restore your nervous system.
- Find a great video course that you feel comfortable with and do it from home.

4. *Eat Good Food and Drink Lots of Water*

- Reduce your sugar intake, and avoid simple carbs (including grains), processed foods, junk food, and deep-fried foods as much as possible.
- Fish is the superfood for recovering mothers; get three servings per week!
- Slow-cooked and pressure-cooked foods like soups and bone broths are fortifying and easy to digest, will speed up your recovery, and can be made in large amounts (enough for two or three extra meals), which will cut down on your cooking time over the course of a week.
- Set up a food roster or a meal train whereby friends and family bring food to you for a few weeks. Or try to get someone to come into your kitchen and prepare a few days' worth of food for you. You'd be surprised how many people will be happy to help when you give them specific instructions—and hopefully they'll clean up afterward, too!
- The best water to drink is genuine spring water. You want at least a half gallon a day and more if you're breastfeeding.

5. *Be Active*

- As long as you've been given the go-ahead by your doctor, find ways to move every day.
- Aim for at least thirty minutes of walking every day. You don't have to do it all at once.
- Do your home-based exercises for your pelvic floor for at least ten minutes every day.

6. Don't Entertain Visitors

- My only somewhat joking advice to new moms about postbirth visitors is "no visitors, only staff"—meaning the only people who should be coming over are those with a job to do (bringing food, bringing supplies, cooking, cleaning, taking the garbage out, watching the baby when you go to yoga, etc.). Outsourcing help (cleaning, babysitting) allows you to sleep and rest.
- Keep a list of things you need and useful to-dos. Remember, your friends and loved ones really do want to help, but they often just don't know how. Tell them where to get your favorite salad, what cleansers to use in the kitchen, that a foot rub would be heavenly, or to bring flowers. If they ask whether you need something, it helps to keep a list so that you can give them specifics!

7. Curb Your Social Media Postings

- It is very important to curb your social media use and to be incredibly selective about what you expose yourself to.
- Limit your exposure to once or twice a day for thirty to sixty minutes max, and *do not use it* outside these times. Switch off all your auto-alerts and subscribed mail lists. Take a hiatus from Facebook. You only want your A team at this time of your life, and online distractions will zap your energy and focus if you try to make decisions about anything other than the immediate task at hand—which is recovering from your depletion.
- Be good to yourself and listen to books on tape; get magazine subscriptions; try out meditation apps; learn a language or take up knitting; make phone calls, not texts. What you want to do is find activities that are nourishing for your soul and pleasing for your spirit.

8. Get Rid of Clutter

- Time to toss! Get ruthless—it feels great. Consider this part of babyproofing and it'll be easy to go through with it.

- Simplify and automate wherever you can. Shop for groceries and baby supplies online and have them delivered. Set up automatic payments on your bills. The less you have to think and make decisions about extraneous stuff, the quicker you will recover.

9. *Be Good to Your Soul*

- Making the time for a short meditation and mantra of gratitude will do wonders for your soul and your spirit. All you need are three minutes of quiet every day to express your feelings.
- Do mindful breathing exercises, with either yoga poses or visualizations, as you learned about in chapter 7. You will always experience deeper relaxation when your exhale is longer than your inhale. A fantastic tool to help with breathing and relaxation is called HeartMath (www.heartmath.com). Five minutes, twice a day can make an enormous difference.

10. *Create Moments for Joy*

- You are amazing! You made a baby! Be proud and thrilled with your body for such an achievement, even when you're still depleted. Your depletion will go away. Your accomplishment will not!
- Put on some music you love, and dance and sing along with your baby. There can never be too much joy in the house.

APPENDIX B

Recommended Reading/ Resources List

FOR THE HOME

Bijlsma, N. *Healthy Home, Healthy Family: Is Where You Live Affecting Your Health?* 3rd Edition (2018).

www.ewg.org

FOR CONCEPTION

Asprey, L. and Asprey, D. *The Better Baby Book: How to Have a Healthier, Smarter, Happier Baby* (2013).

Dittmann, R. *Brighton Baby: A Revolutionary Organic Approach to Having an Extraordinary Child* (2012).

FOR PREGNANCY AND THE FIRST YEAR

Buckley, S. *Gentle Birth, Gentle Mothering: A Doctor's Guide to Natural Childbirth and Gentle Early Parenting Choices* (2009).

Cherry, T. and Hanckel, J. *Eco Parenting: Pregnancy to Year One Guide* (2010).

Gordon, Y. *Birth and Beyond: Pregnancy, Birth, Your Baby, and Family* (2002).

Raffelock, D. et al. *A Natural Guide to Pregnancy and Postpartum Health: The First Book by Doctors That Really Addresses Pregnancy Recovery* (2002).

FOR FOOD

Gedgaudas, N. *Primal Body, Primal Mind: Beyond the Paleo Diet for Total Health and a Longer Life* (2011).

Thanks and Acknowledgments

Caroline—my life partner, the mother of our three fantastic children, and my avatar for this book. It has been deeply moving witnessing your transformation. Thank you for believing so deeply in me, and for embracing our leap of faith together.

To my own mother, Josephine—thank you for showing me through action what gender equality really is. *"Muchos besos, Mama."*

To my father, George, who taught me how, through data and experimentation, to radically question the problem and then how to think differently about it. *"Te echo de menos, Papa."*

Lisa Fitzpatrick—thank you for your incredible support and insights into the world of book writing and into the mythical world of the wise woman. You helped me incredibly early on when I was still trying to make sense of all this, and for that I am deeply grateful.

To the incredible team at GOOP for your support and your belief—a deep heartfelt thank-you to G. P., Elise Loehnen, and Alejandro Junger. Without you this book would still be just an idea.

To my writing and publishing team at Grand Central Publishing—thank you to Karen Moline for your skills, patience, and insights into the art of writing. Thank you to Leah Miller for your support and passion for this important topic.

Big thanks to the exceptional team at The Health Lodge in Byron Bay, who not only share this passion for wellness but who have also inspired and taught me so much about "Mothercare."

An especially big thank-you to Ilse van Oostenbrugge—for your incredible contribution on exercise and movement. Your work as a physiotherapist and as a life coach is groundbreaking, and your wisdom and overview is unparalleled.

Emma McLaughlin and Kristin Zanotti—thank you for your work on the nutrition part of this book. As naturopaths on the frontline, it is only through the work you do assessing and following up on my postnatal clients that it becomes possible to bring the science into very practical usable steps.

Thank you to Dr. Lauren Tober—your work in the community is truly inspiring. Through your combined passions for yoga and psychology you help so many people, and your teachings on gratitude and iRest Yoga Nidra are vital keys to the healing of the planet.

Thank you to Tamar Ben Hur—you truly are a beacon of light for couples navigating the journey of relationships in modern times. Your profound and sometimes radical insights and gentle spiritual perspectives have been a gift for me and have significantly influenced this book on postnatal recovery that covers so much more than just physical well-being.

Thank you to my research team—Quilla Watt, Bron Muir, and Irene Sportel—for your dedication and passion for uncovering the gems of knowledge that have become the backbone of this book.

Phil Baxter—thank you for your insights and your reflections regarding TCM and worldview on maternal health.

Thank you to my community in northern NSW, Australia, for your open-mindedness around new (ancient) alternative ways of practicing medicine, for wanting to be empowered with your health, for seeing and supporting my vision.

Special thanks to Bhavani and Bharat—for your personal support and your belief in me. Thank you for reminding me of the power of transformation.

Bibliography

CHAPTER 1

Deelah, C. "An Overview of Traditional Native American Birth Practices." *Pathways to Family Wellness*, Issue 48 (2015).

Dobson, M. *The Story of Medicine: From Bloodletting to Biotechnology* (2013).

Flood, J. *The Original Australians: Story of the Aboriginal People* (2006).

Gabbe, S. et al. *Obstetrics: Normal and Problem Pregnancies*, 6th edition (2012).

Gedgaudas, N. *Primal Body, Primal Mind: Beyond the Paleo Diet for Total Health and a Longer Life* (2011).

Gordon, Y. *Birth and Beyond: Pregnancy, Birth, Your Baby, and Family* (2002).

Kitzinger, S. *Women As Mothers* (1978).

Maushart, S. *The Mask of Motherhood: How Mothering Changes Everything and Why We Pretend It Doesn't* (1997).

Mukherjee, S. *The Laws of Medicine: Field Notes From an Uncertain Science* (2015).

Pizzorno, J. *The Toxin Solution: How Hidden Poisons in the Air, Water, Food and Products We Use Are Destroying Our Health* (2017).

"Postpartum Beliefs and Practices Among Non-Western Cultures," MCN, *The American Journal of Maternal/Child Nursing*. March/April 2003, Volume 28, Number 2, pages 74–78.

Smith, R. and Lourie, B. *Slow Death by Rubber Duck: How the Toxic Chemistry of Everyday Life Affects Our Health* (2009).

Selin, H. and Stone, P. *Childbirth Across Cultures: Ideas and Practices of Pregnancy, Childbirth, and the Postpartum* (2009).

Silberman, J.; Wang, C.; Mason, S. T.; Schwartz, S. M.; Hall, M.; Morrissette, J. L.; et al. "The Avalanche Hypothesis and Compression of Morbidity: Testing

Assumptions Through Cohort-Sequential Analysis." *PLoS ONE* 10(5) (2015): e0123910. doi:10.1371/ journal.pone.0123910.

Schiebinger, L. "Women's Health and Clinical Trials." *J Clin Invest* 112:973–977 (2003). doi:10.1172/JCI200319993.

CHAPTER 2

Adams Waldorf, K. and Nelson, J. "Autoimmune Disease During Pregnancy and the Microchimerism Legacy of Pregnancy." *Immunol Invest* 2008; 37(5): 631–644. doi:10.1080/08820130802205886.

Brizendine, L. *The Female Brain* (2006).

Creasy, R. and Resnik, R. et al. *Maternal-Fetal Medicine: Principles and Practice,* 7th Edition (2014).

Day, J. et al. *Breast Feeding Naturally,* 2nd Edition. Australian Breastfeeding Association (2004).

Dawe, G; Wei Tan, X.; and Xiao, Z. "Cell Migration from Baby to Mother." *Cell Adhesion & Migration* 2007; 1:1, 19–27

Hoekzema, E. et al. "Pregnancy Leads to Long-Lasting Changes in Human Brain Structure." *Nature Neuroscience* 19 Dec. 2016. doi:10.1038/nn.4458.

Kay, H.; Nelson, M.; and Wang, Y. *The Placenta: From Development to Disease* (2011).

Khashan, A. S.; Kenny, L. C.; Laursen, T. M.; Mahmood, U.; Mortensen, P. B.; Henriksen, T. B.; O'Donoghue, K. "Pregnancy and the Risk of Auto-Immune Disease." *PLoS One* 2011; 6: e19658; PMID: 21611120; DOI: 10.1371/journal.pone.

Knippen, M. "Microchimerism: Sharing Genes in Illness and in Health." *International Scholarly Research Network (ISRN): Nursing Volume.* 2011, Article ID 893819, 4 pages; doi:10.5402/2011/893819.

Lim, R. *After the Baby's Birth: A Complete Guide for Postpartum Women* (2001).

Lim, R. *Placenta: The Forgotten Chakra* (2010).

Loke, Y. *Life's Vital Link: The Astonishing Role of the Placenta* (2013).

Mor, G. et al. *Immunology of Pregnancy* (2006).

Power, M. and Schulkin, J. *The Evolution of the Human Placenta* (2012).

Romm, A. *Natural Health After Birth: The Complete Guide to Postpartum Wellness* (2002).

West, Z. *Natural Pregnancy-Complementary Therapies for Preconception, Pregnancy, and Postnatal Care* (2001).

CHAPTER 3

Brogan, K. *A Mind of Your Own: The Truth About Depression and How Women Can Heal Their Bodies to Reclaim Their Lives* (2016).

Crayton, J. and Walsh, W. "Elevated Serum Copper Levels in Women with a History of Post-Partum Depression." *Journal of Trace Elements in Medicine and Biology*, Volume 21, Issue 1, 14 March 2007, 17–21. doi:10.1016/j.jtemb.2006.10.001.

Deligiannidia, K. and Freeman, M. "Complementary and alternative medicine therapies for perinatal depression." *Best Pract Res Clin Obstet Gynaecol* 2014 January; 28(1): 85–95. doi:10.1016/j.bpobgyn.2013.08.007.

Greenblatt, J. and Brogan, K. *Integrative Therapies for Depression: Redefining Models for Assessment, Treatment, and Prevention* (2016).

Juster, R. P. et al. "Allostatic Load and Comorbidities: A Mitochondrial, Epigenetic, and Evolutionary Perspective." *Development and Psychopathology* 28 (2016), 1117–1146; doi:10.1017/S0954579416000730.

Parker, G., Eyers, K. and Boyce, P. *Overcoming Baby Blues: A Comprehensive Guide to Perinatal Depression* (2014).

World Health Organisation. "Mental Health Aspects of Women's Reproductive Health: A Global Review of the Literature" (2009).

CHAPTER 4

Brownstein, D. *Iodine: Why You Need It, Why You Can't Live Without It*, 4th edition (2009).

Higdon, J. *An Evidence-Based Approach to Vitamins and Minerals: Health Benefits and Intake Recommendations* (2003).

Hollis, B. et al. "Vitamin D Supplementation During Pregnancy: Double-Blind, Randomized Clinical Trial of Safety and Effectiveness." *Journal of Bone and Mineral Research*, Vol. 26, No. 10, October 2011, 2341–2357; DOI: 10.1002/jbmr.463.

Kellerman, G. *Abnormal Laboratory Results* (2006).

Krebs, N. "Zinc Supplementation During Lactation." *Am J Clin Nutr* 1998; 68 (suppl): 509S–12S.

Kyle, C. *Sonic Pathology Handbook: A Guide to the Interpretation of Pathology Tests* (2014).

Lord, R. and Bralley, J. *Laboratory Evaluations for Integrative and Functional Medicine*, 2nd Edition (2008).

Osiecki, H. *The Nutrient Bible*, 9th Edition (2014).

Rheaume-Bleue, K. *Vitamin K2 and the Calcium Paradox: How a Little-Known Vitamin Could Save Your Life* (2012).

Tabrizian, I. *Visual Textbook of Nutritional Medicine* (2012).

WHO. "Guideline: Vitamin A Supplementation in Postpartum Women." World Health Organization, 2011.

CHAPTER 5

Freeman, M. "Complementary and Alternative Medicine for Perinatal Depression." *Journal of Affective Disorders*, 112(1–3) pp1—10 (2009). DOI: http://dx.doi.org/10.1016/j.jad.2008.06.017

Shanahan, C. *Deep Nutrition: Why Your Genes Need Traditional Food* (2008).

Teicholz, N. *The Big Fat Surprise; Why Butter, Meat, and Cheese Belong in a Healthy Diet* (2014).

CHAPTER 6

Brownstein, D. *Overcoming Thyroid Disorders*, 2nd edition (2002).

Buckley, Sarah J. "Executive Summary of Hormonal Physiology of Childbearing: Evidence and Implications for Women, Babies, and Maternity Care." Washington, D.C.: Childbirth Connection Programs, National Partnership for Women and Families, January 2015.

Gordon, M. *The Clinical Application of Interventional Endocrinology* (2007).

Gottfried, S. *The Hormone Cure-Reclaim Balance, Sleep, and Sex Drive; Lose Weight; Feel Focused, Vital, and Energized Naturally with the Gottfried Protocol* (2013).

Weaver, L. *Exhausted to Energized* (2015).

CHAPTER 7

Andrews, L. *The Postpartum Recovery Program: How to Adapt the Ancient Practice of Zuo Yue Zi to Your Patients* (2014).

Farhi, D. *The Breathing Book-Good Health and Vitality Through Essential Breath Work* (1996).

Gardner, Z. *American Herbal Products Association's Botanical Safety* (2013).

Lad, V. *Ayurveda: The Science of Self Healing* (1985).

Lasater, J. *Relax and Renew-Restful Yoga for Stressful Times*, 2nd Edition (2011).

Mills, S. and Bone, K. *The Essential Guide to Herbal Safety* (2005).

Mills E. et al. *Herbal Medicines in Pregnancy and Lactation: An Evidence-Based Approach* (2013).

Ou, H. et al. *The First Forty Days: The Essential Art of Nourishing the New Mother* (2016).

Singh, N. and Gilca, M. *Herbal Medicine-Science Embraces Tradition: A New Insight into Ancient Ayurveda* (2010).

CHAPTER 8

Becker, R. and Selden, G. *The Body Electric; Electromagnetism and the Foundation of Life* (1985).

Braun, L. and Cohen, M. *Herbs and Natural Supplements: An Evidence-Based Guide*, Volume 1 & 2 (2015).

Hansler, R. *Great Sleep! Reduced Cancer! A Scientific Approach* (2008).

Huffington, A. *The Sleep Revolution; Transforming Your Life One Night at a Time* (2016).

Ober, C.; Sinatra, S.; and Zucker, M. *Earthing: The Most Important Health Discovery Ever?* (2010).

Samvat, R. and Osiecki, H. *Sleep, Health, and Consciousness: A Physicians Guide* (2009).

Weed, S. *Wise Woman Herbal for the Childbearing Year* (1986).

CHAPTER 9

Ballantyne, S. *The Paleo Approach-Reverse Autoimmune Disease and Heal Your Body* (2013).

Batmanghelidj, F and Day, P. *The Essential Guide to Water and Salt*, 2nd Edition (2014).

Gundry, S. *The Plant Paradox: The Hidden Dangers in Healthy Foods That Cause Disease and Weight Gain* (2017).

Junger, A. *Clean Gut: The Breakthrough Plan for Eliminating the Root Cause of Disease and Revolutionizing Your Health* (2013).

National Health and Medical Research Council. "Australian Dietary Guidelines." Canberra: National Health and Medical Research Council (2013).

National Health and Medical Research Council Review. "Nutritional Requirements And Dietary Advice Targeted for Pregnant and Breastfeeding Women." Canberra: National Health and Medical Research Council.

Perlmutter, D. *Grain Brain: The Surprising Truth About Wheat, Carbs and Sugar—Your Brain's Silent Killers* (2014).

Perlmutter, D. *Brain Maker: The Power of Gut Microbes to Heal and Protect Your Brain, For Life* (2015).

Pollack, G. *The Fourth Phase of Water: Beyond Solid Liquid Vapour* (2013).

Robinson, R. *Eating On the Wild Side: The Missing Link to Optimum Health* (2013).

Shanahan, C. *Food Rules: A Doctor's Guide to Healthy Eating* (2010).

Smith, J. M. "Survey Reports Improved Health After Avoiding Genetically Modified Foods." *Int J Hum Nutr Funct Med* (2017).

Statham, B. *The Chemical Maze Shopping Companion*, 3rd Edition (2005).

Wrangham, R. *Catching Fire: How Cooking Made Us Human* (2009).

Woodford, K. *Devil in the Milk: Illness, Health, and Politics of A1 and A2 Milk* (2007).

CHAPTER 10

Bershadsky, S. et al. "The Effect of Prenatal Hatha Yoga on Affect, Cortisol, and Depressive Symptoms." *Complementary Therapies in Clinical Practice* Volume 20, Issue 2, May 2014, Pages 106–113

Buttner, M. et al. "Efficacy of Yoga for Depressed Postpartum Women: A Randomized Controlled Trial." *Complementary Therapies in Clinical Practice* .Volume 21, Issue 2, May 2015, Pages 94–100

Chek, Paul. *How to Eat, Move, and Be Healthy*. C.H.E.K Institute (2004).

CHEK Exercise Coach. Advanced Training Program, C.H.E.K Institute (2002).

Chek, Paul. *Equal But Not the Same, Considerations for Training Females.* Volume 1–5

Evenson, K. et al. "Physical Activity Beliefs, Barriers and Enablers Among Postpartum Women." *Journal of Women's Health*, Volume 18, Number 12, 2009; a Mary Ann Liebert, Inc. DOI: 10.1089=jwh.2008.1309

Field, T. "Yoga and Social Support Reduce Prenatal Depression, Anxiety, and Cortisol." *Journal of Bodywork & Movement Therapies* (2013) 17, 397-403

Lee, D. *The Pelvic Girdle: An Integration of Clinical Expertise and Research* (2010).

Magee, D. *Orthopedic Physical Assessment*, 5th Edition (2007).

Mohammadi, F; Malakooti, J; Babapoor, J; Mohammad-Alizadeh-Charandabi, S. "The Effect of a Home-Based Exercise Intervention on Postnatal Depression and Fatigue: A Randomized Controlled Trial." *International Journal of Nursing Practice* (2015); 21: 478–485 doi:10.1111/ijn.12259

Saligheh, et al. "Perceived Barriers and Enablers of Physical Activity in Postpartum Women: A Qualitative Approach." *BMC Pregnancy and Childbirth* (2016) 16:131 DOI 10.1186/s12884-016-0908-x

Sapolsky, Robert M. *Why Zebra's Don't Get Ulcers: An Update Guide to Stress, Stress Related Disease and Coping* (2004).

Spence, N. "The Long-Term Consequences of Childbearing: Physical and Psychological Well-Being of Mothers in Later Life." *Res Aging*. 2008; 30(6): 722–751. doi:10.1177/0164027508322575

Sperstad, J. B.; Tennfjord, M. K.; Hilde, G.; et al. "Diastasis Recti Abdominis During Pregnancy and 12 Months After Childbirth: Prevalence, Risk Factors and Report of Lumbopelvic Pain." *Br J Sports Med* (2016) doi: 10.1136/bjsports-2016-096065

Tseng et al. "A Systematic Review Of Randomised Controlled Trials On The Effectiveness Of Exercise Programs On Lumbo Pelvic Pain Among Postnatal Women." *BMC Pregnancy and Childbirth* (2015) 15:316 DOI 10.1186/s12884-015-0736-4

Vleeming, A. et al. *Movement, Stability, Low Back Pain and the Essential Role of the Pelvis* (1997).

Wang, F. et al. "Long-term Association Between Leisure-time, Physical Activity, and Changes in Happiness: Analysis of the Prospective National Population Health Survey." *Am I Epidemiol* (2012) 176 (12): 1095-1100. DOI: https://doi.org/10.1093/aje/kws199

Zourladani, A. et al. "The Effect of Physical Exercise on Postpartum Fitness, Hormone and Lipid Levels: A Randomized Controlled Trial in Primiparous, Lactating Women." *Arch Gynecol Obstet* (2015) 291:525–530 DOI 10.1007/s00404-014-3418-y

CHAPTER 11

Aron, E. *The Highly Sensitive Person: How to Thrive When the World Overwhelms You* (2016).

Csikszentmihalyi, M. *Flow: The Psychology of Optimal Experience* (1990).

Greenblatt, J. and Brogan, K. *Integrative Therapies for Depression: Redefining Models for Assessment, Treatment, and Prevention* (2016).

CHAPTER 12

Brown, B. *Braving the Wild: The Quest for True Belonging and the Courage to Stand Alone* (2017).

Levine, P. *In an Unspoken Voice: How the Body Releases Trauma and Restores Goodness* (2010).

CHAPTER 13

Callander, M. *Why Dads Leave: Insights and Resources for When Partners Become Parents* (2012).

Crawford, M. *Unlocking the Queen Code: Divine Keys to Reclaiming Your Throne* (2015).

Daedone, N. *Slow Sex: The Art and Craft of the Female Orgasm* (2011).

https://www.children-and-divorce.com/divorce-statistics.html (accessed 17th March 2017)

https://www.heritage.org/marriage-and-family/report/the-effects-divorce-america (accessed 17th March 2017)

http://www.abs.gov.au/People-and-Communities (accessed 17th March 2017)

Institute of Medicine and National Research Council. "Welfare, the Family, and Reproductive Behavior: Report of a Meeting." Washington, D.C.: The National Academies Press (1998). https://doi.org/10.17226/6001.

Maushart, S. *Wifework: What Marriage Really Means for Women* (2001).

Perel, E. *The State of Affairs: Rethinking Infidelity* (2017).

Rosenberg, M. *Nonviolent Communication*, 3rd Edition (2015).

Rubinstein, A. *The Making of Men: Raising Boys to Be Happy, Healthy, and Successful* (2013).

Index

About the Author

Dr. Oscar Serrallach, MBChB, FRACGP, is a doctor of Functional Medicine with a special interest in Postnatal Well-being. Prior to completing his fellowship in General Practice and Family Medicine (Board Certification) in 2010, he worked in Emergency Medicine. His initial studies in Functional Medicine coincided with starting a family, which naturally led him to consider the science through the particular lens of pregnancy, birth, and the postnatal period, observing his own partner and many mothers through his clinical work.

Dr. Serrallach was first to recognize something he termed Postnatal Depletion, describing the broader clinical pattern of many women presenting with symptoms after having children. He has since dedicated his work toward researching this condition and applying the practice of Functional Medicine to help his clients with their recovery. He currently lives near Byron Bay, Australia, with his partner and their three children. *The Postnatal Depletion Cure* is his first book.